The Whole Person Fertility Program^{SM}

The Whole Person FERTILITY Program^{SM}

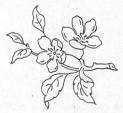

A Revolutionary Mind-Body Process to Help You Conceive

NIRAVI B. PAYNE, M.S.,
AND BRENDA LANE RICHARDSON
FOREWORD BY CHRISTIANE NORTHRUP, M.D.

THREE RIVERS PRESS
NEW YORK

Author's Note

To safeguard my clients' anonymity and their families', biographical details have been changed, as well as any events that contain information that could be used to identify them. In some cases, we have condensed, edited, or combined clients' quotes for the sake of anonymity, clarity, and length. The details of their work in the Whole Person Fertility Program^{SM} and the manner in which clients responded, healed, and conceived has not been altered, for this is the essence of my work.

Published by Three Rivers Press, a division of Crown Publishers, Inc., 201 East 50th Street, New York, New York 10022. Member of the Crown Publishing Group.

Originally published in hardcover by Harmony Books, a division of Crown Publishers, Inc., 1997

Random House, Inc. New York, Toronto, London, Sydney, Auckland www.randomhouse.com

THREE RIVERS PRESS and colophon are trademarks of Crown Publishers, Inc.

Printed in the United States of America

Design by June Bennett-Tantillo

Library of Congress Cataloging-in-Publication Data is available upon request.

ISBN 0-609-80198-8

10 9 8 7 6 5 4 3 2 1

First Paperback Edition

To my dearest children, grandchildren, great-grandchildren, and all the children of the world—big and little. May you know the joy and wonder of realizing your innermost dreams and heartfelt prayers.

—Niravi B. Payne

All my love and thanks to God for my wonderful husband, and our three healthy children. May we continue to benefit from all that I have learned in the creation of this book.

—Brenda Lane Richardson

Contents

Contents

Acknowledgments

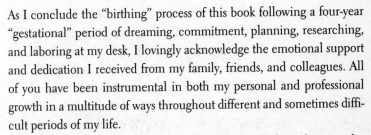

As I conclude the "birthing" process of this book following a four-year "gestational" period of dreaming, commitment, planning, researching, and laboring at my desk, I lovingly acknowledge the emotional support and dedication I received from my family, friends, and colleagues. All of you have been instrumental in both my personal and professional growth in a multitude of ways throughout different and sometimes difficult periods of my life.

To Brenda Lane Richardson, a dedicated and talented writer who gave written shape to my dreams of this book. Thank you for being willing to go up and down the hills and valleys as well as to the top of the mountain in the difficult process of collaboration.

To Dr. Christiane Northrup, for your abiding conviction and moving support of both me and the importance of this work; with deep appreciation for facilitating the publication of the book and writing the beautiful foreword.

To Marcelle Pick, with heartfelt thanks for your genuine trust, enthusiasm, and support of this work and for our meaningful, loving, and growing relationship.

To Leslie Meredith, Editorial Director of Harmony Books, who responded warmly and enthusiastically to my vision and helped bring this work into the world. You have earned my deep and abiding respect for your invaluable editorial assistance as well as your ongoing support for the essence of this book.

To Sherri Rifkin and Laura Wood, two editors whom I deeply appreciate for the long hours they labored to give the manuscript a new shape and their willingness to listen, understand, and respect my views about the book's essence.

To Joanna Burgess, assistant to Sherri, who offered much-appreciated warm, friendly, and efficient assistance during many harried hours.

To Bethany Hays, M.D., a warm and loving thank-you for your much-appreciated "eleventh-hour" willingness to review the manuscript. Your understanding of the book's message was indeed gratifying.

To my daughter Meri, and my son-in-law Jonathan Wallace, who separately and together have been my dearest, most loving, and closest support team in so many ways. Meri has been instrumental in teaching me, as a parent, that one is never "too old" to engage in conscious parenting; that when each is struggling to grow and change inherited generational patterns, a path opens to a loving, healing relationship between mother and daughter. I also want to thank Meri, as a family therapist, for her written contribution to this book. Our relationship has helped me immeasurably in being a healing energy for so many women and their mothers.

To my daughter Bonnee, who is my most provocative teacher on how to stay openhearted to the energy of love. In deep gratitude to her for the privilege of becoming, through her two sons, a great-grandmother with five wonderful great-grandchildren.

To my grandsons, David, Gregg, and Michael, and my granddaughters, Debbie, Lori, and Meredith, for their love, support, wisdom, and delicious, often fun-loving presence in my life.

To Ashley, Landon, Steven, Tyler, and Megan, my treasured great-grandchildren who are teaching me that love and wisdom come in younger people when I take the time to truly listen.

To my loving and supporting sisters, Nancy and Frances, who teach me constantly the sweetness of the word *sister* and how important sisterhood truly is. And to my brother-in-law, Perry, who labored long hours in helping me launch my professional career by producing my first brochure.

To Renia, whose heart and hands lovingly and caringly computerized draft after draft of the manuscript in the interest of excellence. Her understanding, dedication, and support, often into late-night hours, made this book possible.

To Nina Calaman, who brought her expertise, love, and caring to the initial stages of the book's organization.

To Sandy Ferguson, a warm thank-you for your hundreds of hours of invaluable research, which helped to substantiate the book's material.

To Alda Zwilich, who, at eighty-seven, inspired my writing this book many years ago and asked in return only that I acknowledge her presence in my life. She taught me that vitality, energy, and spirit have no age limits.

To my dearest friends and colleagues whose loving, emotional support was invaluable to get me through the tension-filled months of writing and rewriting.

To Rita Kirsch, my friend, colleague, and fellow traveler on this rich journey called life.

To Natalie Rogers, who so caringly helped me design the first ad for my fertility program on the back of a pie plate during a party.

To Dawn Ferber, who for more than thirteen years has been so consistently loving and supportive during some of the very dark and some gloriously light moments in our personal history.

To Dr. Ann Maugeri, my loving friend and colleague and a major part of my health team. Thank you for the long hours you put in doing valued research for the book.

To Gail Owgang, who so warmly came into my life at a crisis moment, to begin the first training program for the Whole Person Fertility Program^{SM}.

To Renee Rosenberg and Linda Millet, who were also part of my loving support team.

To Dr. Roberta Chaplin, my loving friend who shortly after giving form to my initial book proposal left this earth much too soon. I miss you.

And to my many teachers who helped me grow personally and professionally in so many ways.

To Nigrantha, for introducing me to the Fisher-Hoffman process, which literally helped change my life, and for teaching me what being a loving therapist is all about.

To Dr. Daniel Miller, for being the most serious, meaningful, loving, and provocative teacher at the time I was a fledgling human being and therapist.

To my mother's brothers, Jack, Ben, and David, who by their incredible example as leaders instilled in me determination, courage, and above all, a social consciousness.

Last but certainly not the least, with deep gratitude to my mother and father, Jean and Jesse Price, for my life, for without them I wouldn't have been.

— Niravi B. Payne, M.S.

My thanks to Dr. Brenda Wade, Carolyn Waters, Sandy Ferguson, and to Niravi's clients — many of whom I met in the summer of 1995 and who are now proud, loving, and conscious parents.

— Brenda Lane Richardson

Foreword

I first met Niravi Payne in the late 1980s and have been referring patients to her ever since to help them heal fertility and related problems. As a referring physician with intimate knowledge of the medical conditions particular to these patients, I can say with assurance that the success of Niravi's work at helping people heal themselves is incontrovertible proof of the unity of the body, mind, and spirit. Many have gone on to conceive after all other avenues to help solve fertility problems, including very sophisticated technology, have failed. As a witness to Niravi's compassionate and groundbreaking work with fertility, I am honored to have been one of the midwives for the labor and birthing of this book—a volume that contains the missing keys to help so many unlock the mysteries surrounding conception, gestation, labor, and the birth of the new members of our next generation.

Niravi has courageously led the way to the creation of a whole new language and approach to fertility. This language examines how and why unexpressed emotions and unfinished business from childhood affect fertility. But that is just the beginning. Niravi then graciously shows her clients—and now her readers—how the recognition and release of those emotions and the acknowledgment of one's inherent worthiness to live fully can heal her or his relationship with fertility—whether or not a child is ever conceived. Very often when individuals and couples really engage in the transformational work Niravi presents here, they do conceive and give birth to healthy babies.

Though *The Whole Person Fertility Program*^SM is practical and helpful to individuals who are coming to terms with their fertility, it is also a book with a message of extraordinary significance for society in general as we near the end of the twentieth century. Never before have we been more in need of balanced wisdom concerning fertility and children and the need to make our decisions about these issues consciously. And never before have so many women (and men) been critically reevaluating the values and expectations about parenting that they have inherited from society in general and their parents in particular. Countless women, for example, having tasted the joyous gifts of individuation and personal autonomy in the outer world of business and creativity, can no longer go back into the unconscious caretaking roles that have been handed down to them for generations. The sexual revolution of the 1960s, along with birth-control pills and legalized abortion, made it possible for an entire generation to concentrate on career and relationships during the time when, a generation earlier, their mothers were having their first children.

The baby boomers rejected the limitations we saw so clearly in the lives of our mothers and grandmothers, and very often they associated these limitations with childbearing. In so doing, we were at risk of throwing out the baby with the bathwater! The defiant act of saying no to our mothers' (and sometimes fathers') roles and everything for which they stood was a critical step for many. But the pendulum has often swung too far the other way. Many women's lives look successful on the surface, but underneath, we may be overworked, exhausted, and unfulfilled. Science is now discovering that the physiologic states associated with conventional success in the outer world of achievement are often quite different from the physiologic states that favor conception and peaceful gestation.

And all too often the standard dualistic Western approach to fertility difficulties compounds the problem by severing the emotions and the mind from the body. When one believes that one's problems are solely because one's biochemistry is out of whack—and that this is not related to the rest of one's life in any way—one feels victimized by one's body and by one's hormones. And, unfortunately, that very feeling of victimization has physiologic consequences that can adversely affect the endocrine, immune, and central nervous systems even further. Feeling victimized also reinforces the despair that may well have been part of an individual's childhood if that person learned to believe that she (or he) would not be loved and, worse, would be abandoned unless she conformed to artificial standards of behavior or perfection set by her parents and society for how she ought to use her creative energies.

The Whole Person Fertility Program^{SM} is about finding the balance and peace within yourself that so often results in balanced hormones, balanced lives—and sometimes conception. This book will help you heal and make peace with your fertility. It will also help heal your life even when fertility is not an issue. Niravi's work provides a healing balm for all the chaos, turmoil, and grief that many have gone through in their journey toward parenting. It shines with wisdom and hope.

Christiane Northrup, M.D.
Author of *Women's Bodies, Women's Wisdom*

Prologue

Recently, when I lectured to staff members at Mount Sinai Medical Center's Assisted Reproductive Technology Program, I was asked, "How did you get involved in fertility work?" This question encouraged me to look back over the last fifteen years, during which I have personally and professionally experienced the profound effect of uniting the mind and body in the healing process. During these years, I have worked with hundreds of women and men in my fertility practice who talk about their anguish at not being able to conceive. Some have sought me out in an effort to avoid medical intervention, while others continue their medical fertility treatments—particularly when they have come to me upon the recommendation of a physician. And still others opt to discontinue their reproductive medical care during the course of my working with them.

During our sessions, clients come to realize that all of us experience various physical symptoms that offer feedback about how we feel emotionally. Emotions, whether conscious or unconscious, provoke physical responses. Dr. Christiane Northrup has said, "Our bodies mirror our thoughts, emotions and experiences." She and I both believe that memories of painful childhood experiences are "buried deeply in our psyches, densely imbedded in the very tissues of our hearts, breasts, uteruses, and ovaries."[1]

Over the years, I have worked with clients as they emotionally labor to conceive and deliver healthy babies, carry their pregnancies to term when they have had a history of miscarriages, heal if no pregnancy occurs, or seek alternatives to family building. I am grateful to all the women and men I have had the privilege of working with and learning from, and without whom this book could not have been written.

Yet I had no idea that fertility would become my life's work when I received my master's degree from Hunter College in 1975 and began my professional life as a psychotherapist and biofeedback specialist. In working with biofeedback instruments, I saw tangible evidence of what I had always believed in my heart: The mind and emotions have the power to affect the body. As I worked with clients who suffered from ailments ranging from chronic headaches to strokes, I saw how negative thoughts would produce significant physiological changes, as measured by biofeedback instruments.

In 1982, one of my clients, Meryl, a thirty-four-year-old attorney, tearfully told me of her frustration at not being able to conceive. She and her husband, Bernard, thirty-five, also a lawyer, had been trying to have a baby for thirteen years. Meryl cried when she told me, "It hasn't happened to us, but I can't give up my dream of having my own child." I was deeply moved by her, because in the 1940s I had also struggled for two years to conceive. I remember feeling weighed down by self-blame, which is why one of the major elements of the fertility process in this book aims to understand and work through negative, damaging feelings.

The circumstances of my fertility struggle had been somewhat different from Meryl and Bernard's. I was only eighteen in 1942, when my husband, Al, was drafted at the outbreak of World War II. I did not have to face the biological clock running out, but I dreaded the shipping-out deadline that most wives of men in the armed forces faced. The time was emotionally charged for millions of women, for we wondered if we would ever see the men we loved again. Even now, fifty years later, I can still feel the intense pain of those difficult dark days. I followed Al to the army bases where he was stationed, visiting each army hospital along the way, trying to find out why I was not getting pregnant. Doctors could offer no explanation. I felt frustrated, angry, and desperately unhappy.

At the eleventh hour, before my husband was to be shipped out to Europe, he received an overnight pass from Fort Dix for a quick visit to Brooklyn. Miracle of miracles, nine months later, Bonnee Vee Dawn was born on VE-day. Evidently, after two years of struggling to conceive, the tremendous fear that I might never again see my husband alive overrode my unconscious ambivalence about becoming a mother. I eventually gave birth to my other beloved daughter, Meri. But only after I had become involved in fertility work did I begin to understand that what had happened in my family history had contributed to my initial struggle to have a child.

Remembering that difficult time fueled my determination to use my skills as a therapist and biofeedback specialist to help Meryl and Bernard conceive. Our work over the course of a year resulted in the conception of their first child, Alesha, and profoundly affected the future direction of my practice.

Today, whenever I hear their teenage daughter Alesha's voice on the phone, I am reminded that in the process of self-healing and the resolution of painful childhood experiences and family conflicts, it is possible for my clients to create a new life for themselves—a new life together as a couple, a healthy new inner life, and new life in the form of a baby. This is an awesome revelation. It has led me to become totally committed to empowering women and men to take charge of their reproductive lives, their health, and their well-being.

Because of my experiences with many other clients in 1986, I conceived and "birthed" the Whole Person Fertility Program^{SM}, which is located in the Brooklyn Heights area of Brooklyn, New York. Today, this powerful, innovative therapeutic system combines the very latest in mind-body practice and research.

Shortly after I decided to expand my fertility practice, my abiding belief in mind-body healing was sorely tested. In 1988, I was diagnosed with breast cancer, while at the same time six of my clients conceived within one or two weeks of one another. Professionally, these multiple conceptions were an incredible happening, a gratifying reinforcement of the validity and deep truth of my work. I formed a pregnancy support group for my clients, wherein each woman and her mate expressed their dreams as well as their fears and concerns about having a baby. After the births of their babies, we had a "baby cotillion," where the six babies were presented and celebrated. It was one of the most memorable days of my life.

Personally, my struggle with cancer brought me face-to-face with the healing power of mind-body work and taught me that my first priority had to be living consciously. Heeding the wake-up call, I began to see the breast cancer as a large arrow pointing to the need for me to nurture myself and to change the way I related to my family and they to me, thus setting a new direction for my life. I engaged in a lot of self-reflection and emotional-release work as I looked in depth at what was going on personally in my life that had so depressed my immune system and left me undernurtured. The traditional medical treatment I underwent was limited to a lumpectomy, while I also received psychological, nutritional, and chiropractic support, as well as acupuncture treatments. By uniting the power of my mind and body, I have been living cancer-free for nine years.

In the meantime, the first six healthy and thriving newborns were joined by many other babies born to parents in my practice who were committed to their own personal growth, and to conscious parenting. Every year, I receive letters and beautiful photographs of the babies' progress.

The experience of fighting for my own health while at the same time participating in explorations that led to the birth of six new lives made me determined to expand my fertility practice nationally and internationally. It has also led to my writing this book. For years, many of my clients, colleagues, and friends have urged me to make the Whole Person Fertility Program^{SM} and my experiences available to a far larger audience. *The Whole Person Fertility Program*^{SM} grows out of my concern for the health and well-being of the current generation and future generations whose lives will be deeply affected by the decisions we make today regarding our reproductive lives.

Introduction: The Mind-Body Connection in Reproduction

If you have been frustrated in your attempts to conceive, this book can help you. If you have suffered the terrible sadness and disappointment of a miscarriage or a series of miscarriages, this book can help you, too. If you have undergone—or are undergoing—medical fertility treatments, this book can improve the conditions for their success. If your husband or mate has a low sperm count or your biology seems to be unreceptive to his sperm, the program in this book can help you both. This program addresses and helps you resolve a number of other problems that can affect fertility and prevent conception.

The Whole Person Fertility Program[SM] presents a revolutionary mind-body approach to conceiving consciously. The process of conscious conception entails a willingness to understand the origin of the negative messages that your mind is communicating to your body. Your body communicates to you through physical symptoms, particularly as reproductive difficulties. Conscious conception means that you deliberately use your mind to translate the physical symptoms, particularly blocks to conception, by identifying and releasing deeply held unexpressed emotions. I recognize that there are certain physical conditions that can prevent a pregnancy (for instance, certain STDs and some environmental pollutants may cause permanent damage to reproductive organs), but I have found that the vast majority of reproductive difficulties are responsive to mind-body fertility therapy. This approach will help you whether or not you are working with a medical fertility specialist. In fact, the processes and messages of this book can decisively increase the effectiveness of fertility treatments.

As you read *The Whole Person Fertility Program*^{SM}, I will guide you through a process that considers how your family history and childhood experiences have affected your reproductive system and your ability to become pregnant. In the past fifteen years as a fertility therapist, I have worked with hundreds of clients who initially viewed their difficulties in conceiving as solely a medical problem. In broadening their views and allowing themselves to explore some troublesome and even sometimes painful issues of their personal lives and histories, they were able to address and heal from past problems that had continued to affect them over the years. Healing childhood wounds is not only a way to reclaim your reproductive rights, which is vital for women seeking to become pregnant and to hold a baby to term, but is also a way to heal many other aspects of your life.

This work is effective because the Whole Person Fertility Program^{SM} recognizes that our state of mind and physiological processes are interconnected. Harvard Medical School has an endowed mind-body chair. The physician who currently heads this program, Dr. Herbert Benson, one of the pioneers of mind-body medicine, uses the metaphor of a three-legged stool to represent the proper balance needed in medicine. One leg is pharmaceuticals, the other is surgery, and the third is mind-body medicine, what people can do for themselves.

Because your body constantly is influenced by your emotions, thoughts, and beliefs, which manifest themselves physically, your life story becomes your biology. Mind-body talk is the "language of your fertility," which only you can translate to allow your mind and body to communicate harmoniously. Mind-body counselor Barbara Levine writes, "The guiding light of the body is the mind. Recognizing the connection between language and wellness enables you to expand your control of the healing process. The language connection consists of the thoughts, words, imaginings, mental pictures, and emotions that stimu-late illness and wellness."[1]

Your grief, sadness, disappointments, anger, and other negative experiences show up as symptoms and ailments in your body. After translating the messages behind these symptoms, the challenge then is to change the life situations to which your mind-body is responding negatively.

Often when I suggest that there is a connection between the mind and body, some of my clients will question, "Are you blaming me for my fertility problems?" On the contrary, I want to emphasize that you, your body, and your partner are not to blame if you have not become pregnant. Becoming aware of emotional issues involved in conception and understanding the messages in your family system about sexuality, conception, pregnancy, birthing, and parenting can *free* you from damaging conscious and unconscious self-blame. As you deepen your awareness of the vital connections between how you feel—your inher-ited belief systems; your learned, conditioned responses to the circum-stances, people, and events in your life—and what happens in your body—you can influence your ability to conceive by making changes in your *life.*

The Mind-Body Connection in Reproduction

We have entered an era in which scientific studies have validated that mind and body are interconnected and interdependent. Our thoughts, images, sensations, and feelings interact constantly to trigger responses in our bodies. Although scientists once assumed the mind resided solely in the brain, most now recognize that the mind is connected both phys-ically and chemically with every cell in the body. The mind, in fact, is the aggregate of our capacities for consciousness, memory, and percep-tion. In this book, I'll use the term *mind-body* to mean the intercon-nectedness of our emotional and physical states.

The ongoing dialogue between our thoughts and feelings triggers responses in our bodies that lead to chemical, hormonal, and neurological changes that can throw off the delicate balance of the hormonal system involved in reproduction. Even if our conscious mind is not aware of what we are feeling about an event, person, or experience, the body registers our emotional reactions, which can manifest themselves in the form of reproductive problems, as well as many other physical symptoms. This concept has long been part of our everyday speech; consider phrases such as "You are a pain in my neck"; "She died of a broken heart"; and "It made me sick to my stomach." Although we use these commonplace phrases repeatedly, many people are still largely unaware of the vital connection between how we feel emotionally and how we feel physically.

Suppressed emotions do express themselves in everyone's body, but in a multiplicity of ways: backaches, colds, allergies, gastrointestinal distress, ulcers, chronic fatigue or anxiety, heart attacks, and cancer, and even frequent accidents and professional derailments. While an increase in reproductive problems among women and men today may be partially attributable to environmental factors, a body of research indicates that emotional conflict can upset the healthy functioning of bodily systems. Your work with this book will help you understand why your particular conflicts affect you reproductively, so you can bring about the necessary changes in your life.

Many people resist the idea that there is an interrelationship between the mind and body, because, perhaps without even realizing it, they don't want to feel the pain of a particular experience. The reason we disassociate from our bodies in the first place is so that we don't have to feel physically or emotionally uncomfortable or take any responsibility for changing our lives. Noting the interplay of emotions and physical responses, Dr. Lewis Mehl writes, "From birth, we are obviously inseparable from our bodies...our...unique and individual form of expression....Some people who feel very separate from their body...may react adversely to the psychophysiological view of [reproductive problems]."[2] You might not realize that you are saying yes to having a baby on an intellectual level but no to pregnancy because of your body's storehouse of painful memories.

Emotional conflicts can arise in the form of family secrets we unknowingly keep from ourselves—from our conscious minds—through repressed memories. We often don't allow ourselves to think about certain painful things. However, we can't keep secrets from our bodies. The body remembers what the mind wants to forget. As Dr. Christiane Northrup cautions, "If we do not work through our emotional distress, we set ourselves up for physical distress because of the biochemical effect that suppressed emotions have on our immune and endocrine systems."[3]

Studies have confirmed that your emotions can affect your delicately balanced hormonal system, which controls ovulation, spermatogenesis, and pregnancy. As Dr. Frank Minirth writes in *The Power of Memories*, "Bad, painful memories are not stored in the same way as happy, pleasant memories. The painful memories are stored behind a protective wall which prevents easy access so that they do not continue to hurt constantly."[4] Unresolved painful memories express themselves in the body in the form of physical symptoms.

The Science of Emotion, Memory, and Physiological Responses

As you explore the complex interaction of psychological and physiological factors involved in reproduction, the "Mind-Body Intercommunication Map in Reproduction: How Our Hormonal System Is Affected by Negative Emotional States" (see page 6) will be very helpful in understanding how your emotional reactions affect your ability to conceive. The map outlines the flow between stored negative emotional memories (Negative Family-Talk); their impact on how you feel about yourself (Negative Self-Talk); and the physiological reactions they trigger throughout the body (Mind-Body Talk).

Dr. Larry Cahill, a researcher at the Center for Neurobiology of Learning and Memory at the University of California at Irvine, has found that the brain has two memory systems, one for ordinary information and one for emotionally charged information. His work helps identify what makes emotional moments register in our bodies with such potency.[5]

MIND-BODY INTERCOMMUNICATION MAP IN REPRODUCTION℠

How Our Hormonal System Is Affected by Negative Emotional States

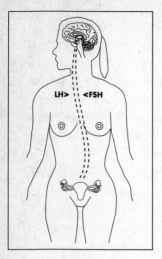

Note: A two-way arrow indicates the circular nature of mind-body interactions—each element affecting the other in both directions.

MIND-BRAIN

- The emotional brain records and stores every experience, from in utero through adulthood—consciously or unconsciously—in long- and short-term memory banks.

- The stored experiences and messages from family patterns of thoughts, feelings, beliefs, and behaviors affect—positively and negatively—how we feel about ourselves.

- Negative emotional responses to these experiences (fear, anger, anxiety, depression, for example) are transformed by the brain into biochemical and electrical messages, which are then released directly into the bloodstream and transmitted to the hypothalamic/pituitary/gonadal axis, hormonally responsible for reproduction.

HYPOTHALAMUS

- Located under the cerebral cortex of the brain.

- Extremely sensitive major pathway, serving as a relay station for transmitting emotionally induced messages from the brain to our reproductive organs.

- Responsible for regulating the delicate balance of hormones to induce the maturation of germ cells (i.e., ovum and sperm).

- In response to emotional distress, it may either cease to secrete or release depleted GnRH messenger chemicals that it sends to the pituitary gland.

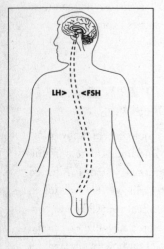

PITUITARY GLAND

- Tiny master gland located at the base of the brain takes its cue from the hypothalamus. The depleted GnRH negatively affects the release of LH and FSH—the two most important hormones in reproduction—thereby interfering with ovulation and spermatogenesis.

- Negative hormonal communication along the hypothalamic/pituitary/gonadal axis is key to the most common cause of difficulty in conception—disruption of ovulation.

REPRODUCTIVE PROBLEMS

WOMEN

- Hypothalamic amenorrhea
- Anovulation (suppression of ovulation)
- Excessive menstrual bleeding
- Depressed progesterone levels
- Fallopian tubal spasms
- Luteal phase defects
- Thinning of endometrial lining

MEN

- Disrupted spermatogenesis: low sperm count, poor motility, abnormal sperm development
- Depressed testosterone levels
- Impotency

These memory systems operate on the same premise as the body's alert system, which primes the body to react to life-threatening situations. Although the primary goal of the fight-or-flight response is to help humans respond to danger, it can also be activated by anger—whether we are conscious of this anger or whether it exists on the unconscious level, where it is stored in our memory banks. Daniel Goleman writes, "A universal trigger for anger is the sense of feeling endangered. Endangerment can be signaled not just by an outright physical threat but also, as is more often the case, by a symbolic threat to self-esteem or dignity; being treated unjustly or rudely, being insulted or demeaned, being frustrated in pursuing an important goal. These perceptions act as the instigating trigger for a limbic surge that has a dual effect on the brain."[6] One part of this surge generates a quick rush of energy in which the body is readied "for a good fight or a quick flight, depending on how the emotional brain sizes up the opposition."[7] Another part of this surge generates a longer-lasting reaction for hours and even days with more physical consequences to our mind-body when we neither fight nor flee. Repressing our feelings, particularly anger, creates an emotional state in which "anger builds on anger."[8] What we are now realizing is that repressing our feelings, particularly anger, has serious psychological and physiological consequences. Negative voices lose their power when we are willing to hear them.

Daniel Goleman states, "The fact that the thinking brain grew from the emotional brain reveals much about the relationship of thought to feelings; there was an emotional brain long before there was a rational one."[9] Emotional responses such as fear, anger, anxiety, and so on are transformed into biochemical messengers and transmitted via nerve fibers traveling from the brain through the spinal cord to the hypothalamus/pituitary control center. This center is extremely sensitive to both emotional and physical tension-filled biochemical messages.

Inherited beliefs and attitudes, what I call "generational family mind talk" and personal beliefs and attitudes, called negative "self-talk"—the foundations for our emotional memories and responses—"have a direct causative effect on the endocrine (hormonal) system via the direct stimulation of the amygdala and its interrelationship with the hypothalamus and the parts of the brain involved in emotions."[10]

You will notice that the map on page 6 also demonstrates how negative self-talk leads to feelings of depression. Dr. Kate Lapane, assistant professor of research at Brown University, and several other researchers found that women who had preexisting feelings of depression—for which the women had not sought clinical help—were twice as likely to have reproductive problems as women who did not report a history of depression. "Before this study," Dr. Lapane said recently in a telephone interview, "the focus of most research in this area was on the depression that was caused as a consequence of infertility. The results of our study indicate that depression may be antecedent to fertility problems." Dr. Lapane explained that she believes the women in her study were struggling with depression that was tied to unresolved childhood issues. Another study, which focused on women who are depressed and undergoing in vitro fertilization (IVF) and embryo-transfer procedures, found that these women had less than 50 percent fewer successful pregnancies than women undergoing IVFs who did not have histories of depression.[11]

In my experience, a number of women with whom I have worked, who were in a depressed emotional state when they entered therapy, were able to work through the depressive state as they connected their feelings to their cause.

A New Language of Fertility

Today, many women thirty-five or older who are conscious of diet and exercise and are healthier than their mothers were at the same age are being unfairly called "perimenopausal," a term formerly used only to describe much older women. In chapter 2, "Who Says I Am Too Old?", I challenge dictums that declare millions of vibrant, healthy women "old." I call this sort of medical diagnosis "the language of futility," which also includes common terms that are applied to women, such as *unexplained infertility, secondary infertility, premature ovarian failure,* and *cervical incompetency*; the labeling of a woman or her eggs as "too old"; as well as terms that are applied to a man, such as *faulty* or *poor sperm production* and *poor motility*. Negative words and labels attributable to reproductive issues represent a limited view of the multiple factors of the mind-body connection to conception. I view these diagnoses as the beginning, not the end, of a couple's quest for a baby. I have worked with many couples who were labeled "infertile" by the medical system but who eventually conceived and gave birth to healthy babies.

This book gives you a new way of looking at what causes fertility problems, and a new vision of how you can see yourself as a fertile being. For that reason, you will find that I use the word "infertility" only within the context of a quote from another author's work or when I place quotation marks around it—to call attention to its potentially damaging effect. Usually, if a woman does not conceive over a given period of time, she is labeled "infertile," which can be incredibly injurious to her self-esteem—and to her fertility, which is often intact and functional. Hearing such hurtful terms can only exacerbate the negative feelings you may have carried since you began to experience difficulty in conceiving, as well as compound the fertility problem itself.

I prefer to use the expression "language of fertility," which is positive and healing. *Webster's* defines the word *fertility* as a broader process of nature, an abundant, fruitful, and ongoing life process. Describing fertility strictly in medical terms as the ability to conceive and give birth ignores a woman's unique human characteristics. Fertility in its truest meaning reflects a vital sense of oneself and a relationship with the rest of the world whether one conceives or not. I call my process the Whole Person Fertility Program[SM] because I have experienced the positive effect on clients who, in exploring the unity of mind and body, have opened themselves to the possibility of conception. The Whole Person Fertility Program[SM] can help you: (1) explore your conscious and unconscious childhood memories and experiences, and the family beliefs that have influenced your thoughts, attitudes, feelings, and behavior about menstruation, sexuality, conception, pregnancy, and childbirth; (2) work through long-forgotten painful memories with emotional-release techniques that allow you to connect with the vital energy that is held back by your past, which is necessary for successful pregnancies; (3) listen to what your body is saying; and (4) become aware of what you are truly feeling, not what you may have learned as a child that you should be feeling.

To develop a "Whole Person" perspective, we need to view ourselves now as fertile beings, uniting our mind and body in the process of seeking to conceive a child. The problem for many of us is that most of our lives we have been accustomed to looking outside of ourselves for healing what ails us inside. *The Whole Person Fertility Program*^{SM} will help you resolve the age-old split between "it's all in your mind" and the equally damaging view "it's all in your body." Many of us are unaware of the connection between our bodies and our emotions. These views can leave us feeling that something is wrong with us emotionally and that we are to blame, or we turn to drugs and surgery as a cure-all for the "sick" body. Drugs and surgery may at times be necessary, but an overreliance on them has resulted in our not trusting the wisdom of our bodies, even when they send messages in the form of reproductive problems.

If we are willing, however, to listen to our bodies' symptoms and think of them as messages and wake-up calls about our lives, we can begin to make the necessary changes to live in healthier ways— emotionally and physically. As you view the difficulties you have in conceiving as an outgrowth of learned childhood experiences and response—and not as a personal inadequacy—you will open yourself to the possibility of conception. In this way, you can begin to approach the journey toward having a baby as one of commitment to your own growth and development.

By no means am I suggesting that you put off or discontinue your medical fertility treatments. In fact, I work with many patients who are actively pursuing such treatments. Dr. Christiane Northrup, who wrote the foreword to this book, and several other physicians often refer their fertility patients to me. These doctors and I believe that through a close collaboration among physical and mental health practitioners, healing can combine medical and holistic treatments.

Although many fertility clinics now include psychological care units, they basically offer only screening and support services for their patients who are undergoing medical fertility treatments. Ideally, these services need to be offered to women and men who do not elect to have medical treatment. I hope this book will heighten the awareness of the public and of medical fertility specialists of the need to explore the pre-existing emotional and family issues that affect millions of women and men. While this book should enhance the success of medical fertility procedures, its main goal is to enrich the emotional and physical lives of those eagerly seeking to conceive or heal if no pregnancy occurs.

Success Beyond Numbers

We need a new definition of "success" rather than always labeling a process or a person as a "failure" if no pregnancy occurs. When I am asked about my success rate, I choose not to engage in the numbers game. Although many healthy babies have emerged from my work, the processes I have developed enable clients to heal generational wounds as they learn to accept themselves in a spirit of wholeness and self-love, whether or not they conceive. They can then move on to consider alternatives, such as adoption, donor eggs, or no children at all with calmer, peaceful, and more open minds.

Using This Book

The Whole Person Fertility Program^{SM} is not a magic pill. It requires hard work, commitment, and patience, but it reaps tremendous benefits. You may need to commit several months of work to the Whole Person Fertility Program^{SM}. Clients generally work with me for periods ranging from several months to a year or more, depending upon their issues, needs, and willingness to pursue an investigation into key areas of their lives. I understand that it can be very frustrating for you not to have a specific time frame, but it may help you to remind yourself of the parable of the two farmers. Farmer A and Farmer B meticulously plant their seeds a half-inch apart, row after row. They look up at the sky. They feel that the sun's rays are warm and penetrating and that the wind is blowing. All looks quite favorable for a good crop. They go back into their farmhouses. The next morning, Farmer A goes out, patiently waters the soil, adds fertilizer, looks up at the sky, prays a bit for rain, and then completes the rest of her chores. On the other hand, Farmer B rushes out in the morning and runs up and down the rows where she had planted her seeds, thinking that miraculously, overnight, at least some shoots should be visible. She then proceeds to dig up the soil, looking at the seeds, saying, "Did you take? Did you take?" You obviously know which farmer will have a bumper crop. More important, which farmer are you? Are you willing to become truly committed to and involved in the work of your garden, cultivating it with patience and thoroughness? The harvest—a word that applies to any activity or endeavor to which you are committed—cannot be hastened. This idea of not rushing the process certainly applies to your work healing yourself and reaping its rewards.

It is also an emotionally intense process, and you'll need to draw on a good deal of your strength, courage, and determination to become aware of the emotionally based issues that can affect your fertility and to live more consciously. As you work through this book, you will find that some of the techniques and exercises may evoke strong emotional reactions. For that reason, you may find it helpful to consider finding a therapist to work with or joining a support group. Additionally, having a close friend or relative as well as your mate read this book along with you will support and further your exploration.

While this book mainly addresses fertility issues from a woman's perspective, I have included a special chapter that is addressed directly to men and discusses men's physical and emotional reproductive challenges. The Whole Person Fertility Program^{SM} is about healing, whether you are a woman or a man. In my practice, I treat women and men individually or as couples, because no matter who has been diagnosed with a reproductive difficulty, both parties are generally involved and can benefit from this process. I strongly urge that as partners on the road to conception, your mate read the entire book and engage in the process along with you, or, at the very least, read chapter 10, which discusses how these issues can affect the reproductive lives of men. Throughout the book, I suggest that your partner complete certain exercises. Your joint participation in these exercises will enhance greatly your chances for success as well as enhance your relationship.

Throughout *The Whole Person Fertility Program*^{SM}, in order to illustrate these issues, I have included prototypical stories that are based on an amalgam of clients' experiences. These stories may trigger the recall of your own memories, causing you to reexamine childhood experiences, which you may or may not have connected to your difficulty in conceiving. The questions and exercises are designed to help you make healing connections through discovering essential truths about your family history that may be affecting your reproductive life today. You can engage in the same highly effective processes and exercises that I have developed to help my clients heal and consciously conceive. In order to get the full benefits of the program, you will need to complete several exercises in the sections entitled "Self-Exploration" and those in chapter 5, as well as reflect on and answer the questions posed in the "For Your Consideration" sections.

Although many healthy babies have emerged from my work, the mind-body process also enables clients to heal generational wounds, whether or not they have a baby. Most important, they learn to accept themselves in a spirit of wholeness and self-love. As you identify and resolve the current effects of your childhood experiences, you will free up your own inner strength and sense of personal power to take charge of your reproductive life more effectively. By participating in the mind-body fertility process, you can gain a new, unique perspective on the inner dynamics of conceiving, carrying a baby to term, and having a successful labor and delivery process.

PART ONE

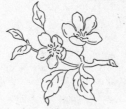

*How Social Forces Have
Affected Your Fertility*

ONE

....

Why So Many Baby Boomers Are Experiencing Fertility Problems

As adults, baby boomers have taken part in the most profound social changes in history—including the sexual revolution, which changed the course of reproductive life familiar to their parents and thirty thousand generations before them. An estimated 90 percent of my clients are baby boomers who put off having children until they felt the time was right for them. They postponed marriage until they achieved financial security and found a partner they loved. They delayed pregnancy until they felt mature enough to forge an emotionally satisfying relationship that could provide them and their children with a nurturing atmosphere.

An estimated ten million American couples (that is, one in six couples, or 15 percent), many of them baby boomers—and a growing number of younger people between the ages of twenty-two and twenty-eight—are experiencing the profound disappointment of not being able to conceive. Others are additionally frustrated after undergoing expensive yet unsuccessful reproductive medical treatments. Throughout this book, you will learn to explore how your intensely personal and unique childhood history has affected you reproductively. As an essential part of that process, it is important to examine how your decisions concerning career, marriage, and childbearing may have been affected by the social issues that differ from generation to generation.

I will never forget one young woman who looked at me rather wistfully and said, "Given my difficulties in conceiving, maybe I should have done what your generation did—have my babies first." As someone who witnessed the sweeping social changes that have taken place from the Great Depression through World War II to the present, I celebrate women of your generation—and women now in their twenties—for having the courage to change the status quo. In my generation, which is the generation of many of my clients' parents, we did not question whether we truly wanted to be married or to have babies right away. The men were being sent off to war, and the women did not know if they would ever return. Young wives during and right after World War II contributed to the postwar skyrocketing birth rate that gave rise to the baby boomer generation. Many women and men put on hold their fondest dreams of study, careers, or creative pursuits to get married and have children. This was considered the natural order of life, and for women, few other options were available or socially acceptable.

Although baby boomer women are like no other women before them, what most women today do not realize is that their lives and their choices are more like those of their grandmothers than their mothers. In the 1930s, we, like you today, were told we could grow up, have careers, and be wives and mothers at the same time. Before the Depression, the United States was viewed as a land of opportunity for women as well as men. Women made up 40 percent of the students in institutions of higher learning, versus 22 percent in England.[1]

But life for women of my generation—and perhaps your mother's—began to change radically as a result of the Great Depression, which caused rampant economic and emotional deprivation. When the United States entered World War II in 1941, five million women were drawn into the workforce to replace men serving in the armed forces[2]—and millions more worked full-time in war-related volunteer activities. Government-sponsored day-care centers were opened to facilitate women's transition to being working women, allowing many women to experience economic independence for the first time. Rosie the Riveter became a symbol of the new and powerful working woman.

The postwar years that followed were marked by a period of great hope and prosperity as the Gross National Product doubled—but for women, this period was marked by a series of retrogressive trends. Postwar conformity spurred traditionalists to tout the return of the ultrafeminine woman as the ideal.

By war's end, the pent-up demand for a normal life led to an era of "ultra-domesticity," a period when home and hearth were considered a woman's greatest calling, according to historian Sylvia Hewlett, whose research provided me with a better understanding of the mothers of baby boomers.[3] Even if your mother didn't want that lifestyle, the emotional and social pressures would have forced her to give up her dreams of a career and other creative pursuits. The gutsy, emancipated women of the 1930s and the war years had to be redefined if they were to create the "home and hearth" for the men. As a consequence, despite considerable advances made by women in the first half of this century, in the late 1940s and 1950s, life again changed dramatically for American women.

To fully understand and appreciate the tremendous psychological, social, and political significance of the baby boomers' groundbreaking changes—which eventually affected the reproductive efforts of millions of women and men—it's crucial to look at the impact on their lives and the lives of their parents of what has been considered one of the most repressive periods in American history: the late 1940s and 1950s. Placing this history into context can help us understand why the baby boomers eventually rebelled and said no to childbearing in their early twenties. Recognizing, of course, that all of history is interconnected and interdependent and prior periods have produced significant changes in the lives of American women from the early pioneering days on, we will concentrate on the postwar time period as the most significant one affecting the baby boomers.

With the soldiers returning home and anxious to be reinstated in their jobs, women were strongly encouraged by American policy makers to resign from the workplace to make way for male workers; many of those who did not were fired. Despite national protests by women's groups, federal subsidies ended for day-care centers that had opened during World War II. A major piece of legislation that aided the domestication of the American woman was the passage of the G.I. Bill of Rights, which literally encouraged early marriage and procreation by providing free college tuition, vocational training, subsistence allowances that increased by 50 percent if one had dependents, and low-cost mortgages that allowed couples to move their families into suburban enclaves—located too far away from cities to make it affordable for women to work. This initiated a trend of fathers riding the commuter trains to the city, which left little time for their families.

This was a time when some high schools taught girls how to select husbands. The birth rate doubled—76 million Americans were born between 1946 and 1964. Not surprisingly, the enrollment of women in college plummeted. Hewlett writes in a tone of outrage, "No wonder there were fewer women lawyers, engineers, and college professors in the fifties than in the thirties."[4] These social conditions explain why so many of my baby boomer clients' grandmothers were college educated and involved in local politics, businesses, schools, civic organizations, and so on, while several of those same clients' mothers were homemakers. There were, of course, many college-educated mothers of baby boomers, but like so many other women of the fifties, most reluctantly yielded to pressure about when and whom to marry, and when to have children.

For the first time in U.S. history, educated women were expected to and encouraged to devote their prime years and expend their best energies on family and home. This was the era of political repression and conformity, which glorified full-time mothers as "true patriots" and declared that no career was as important as that of homemaker and mother. The average age for women to marry dropped to twenty in 1950, down from twenty-three in the 1920s and 1930s. No other industrial country had such an early average age for marriage at the time. Sex was for procreation, with marriage as a prerequisite. While in Europe women gained ground in the 1950s, in the United States they lost considerable turf in terms of education and career, with fewer female graduates then than during the Depression in the 1930s. Women earned 10 percent of doctoral degrees, compared to 17 percent in the 1920s and

'30s; and the proportion of law degrees going to women declined from 6 percent in the 1930s to less than 3 percent in 1959.

The expectations of men also underwent change. Fathers of baby boomers were encouraged to shape their self-identities and self-images in familial and parental roles. The roles were clearly defined: The male is the breadwinner; the female is a full-time mother at home. Fatherhood was considered an important responsibility and evidence of maturity, patriotism, and citizenship. Women who wanted to continue working were seen as a threat to their husbands' "manhood," defined by his role as the breadwinner, and were vilified for "abandoning," or "neglecting," their children. Any woman who consciously or unconsciously avoided the "natural" female role of wife and mother was labeled neurotic and unfit for parenthood. As a consequence, many of these mothers felt intense frustration in their lives, stuck, as many were, in marriages that were often unrewarding, and they felt unable to break away due to economic and emotional dependency. It is not surprising, then, that the level of depression and alcoholism among women rose, inspiring the writing of the *Feminine Mystique* by Betty Friedan. She placed the depression and malaise that these women were feeling in a larger context and confirmed that they were neither sick nor crazy. The *Feminine Mystique* made sense out of their feelings. This was the life to which millions of baby boomers said a resounding no.

Joan, forty-three, a political consultant, admitted that "I followed in my father's footsteps—out the door and away from my mother's life. I was desperately afraid of being like her. She was terribly unhappy, hated her life, and died of a heart attack when she was only forty-eight. When I was thirty, I was shocked to learn that she'd finished college. My dad has a law degree from Yale, and there had always been evidence of that around our house. But I knew little about my mother's education because Daddy always answered for her." Amy, another baby boomer client, explained that her mother had made it quite clear to her daughters that her dream of going to New York as a prima ballerina was destroyed by getting married and having children.

The message to Joan, Amy, and millions of baby boomer women

was clear: You can either have a life or get married and have children. This idea caused deep-seated emotional conflicts between the reality of their own home life versus the ideal but unreal television version of home life. Shows such as *Father Knows Best* and *Ozzie and Harriet* portrayed the happy, compliant housewife with a frilly apron and high heels as the quintessential, perfect mother. The production of TV sets rose from six thousand in 1946 to seven million in 1953, bringing fantasyland into our living rooms. The families portrayed were intact, white, and middle class and the parents were wise, particularly the fathers.

In their real homes, many baby boomer children witnessed their mothers' discontent. Some mothers of baby boomers resented their daughters' rejection of them as role models and punished them out of jealousy. Others encouraged their daughters to pursue their careers and have babies later.

Karen, thirty-eight, an elementary school teacher, recalled that her mother encouraged her to get an education, often pointing out that without a career, a woman had, in her words, "nothing to fall back on." Karen said, "My mother had no life of her own, only bits and pieces of my father's life and her children's. She had to sneak, beg, and manipulate to get around my father. I swore I'd never ever accept her life." This expresses the sentiment of the vast majority of my clients. Emotional discontent prompted women to repudiate their mothers' lives. Although some social observers have blamed the feminist movement for the baby boomers' delay in childbearing, in my view, this political movement was conceived in response to the pain, anger, and frustration women in the 1960s saw in their mothers' lives.

Journalist Ann Taylor Fleming writes, "The roots of my personal journey away from motherhood and that of my contemporaries had begun much earlier in our own childhood home."[5] Surely it is no coincidence that the generation that internalized their mothers' discontent and rebelled against their mothers' lives is the same generation struggling in unprecedented numbers to conceive. As we will explore in depth in chapter 3, this radical breaking away caused an emotional disconnection from mother that seriously affected the later efforts of baby boomer women to conceive.

The Sexual Revolution

The repressive and conformist society of the 1950s gave way to the expressive counterculture values of the 1960s and 1970s. Against the turbulent backdrop of Woodstock (the ultimate "be-in"); civil rights struggles; mounting anti–Vietnam War/antiestablishment movements; Kent State killings; and the murders of President Kennedy, Robert Kennedy, and Martin Luther King, Jr., the boomers attempted to forge new identities that were unlike their parents'. As the Beatles sang, "Give peace a chance," many of the boomers chanted, "We shall overcome." As part of this process, tens of millions of boomers left organized religion as part of their dropout from the culture of their parents. It is in the midst of these emotionally charged times that two major social phenomena occurred which truly revolutionized the lives of women forever.

The development in the 1960s of inexpensive, reliable, and widely distributed oral contraceptives and the legalization of abortions in the 1970s enabled women to avoid repeating their mothers' destinies. The pill allowed women a sense of sexual freedom, and abortions were a safety net that protected many from their fear of having babies early in life and becoming trapped in marriage and motherhood without an education or the ability to make a living. Paving the way for a sexual revolution, the pill "disconnected fear of pregnancy from the pursuit of sexual pleasure," writes Bernard Asbell, author of *The Pill: A Biography of the Drug That Changed the World*.[6] This mass alteration of a reproductive pattern that had existed for thousands of generations had far-reaching cultural implications.

Baby boomers were among the first generation of women to leave home to enter college. Many felt a sense of newfound freedom. Sex for procreation gave way to sex for recreation. The sexual revolution, according to Ann Taylor Fleming, "decisively nudged us further along our path away from motherhood as we evolved into the eroticized generation."[7] Although many steadfastly clung to the moral codes they had learned in their homes, by the late 1960s, the number of women who reported engaging in premarital sex had doubled.[8] According to a 1994 article in *Time*, "The percentage of adults who have racked up twenty-one or more sex partners is significantly higher among the fortysomething boomers than among other Americans."[9] In my experience, although the behavior of so many changed radically during a relatively short period, the beliefs and attitudes many learned from their parents were powerful enough to create considerable conflict and affect their views of themselves as sexual beings. Relaxed sexual attitudes allowed for physical but not emotional freedom. One indication of this is that despite the determination of so many of my clients to lead drastically different lives, they as well as millions of other baby boomer women still became pregnant at about the same age as their mothers. But because of the legalization of abortions, they could, for the first time in history, exercise a reproductive choice.

Most women and men don't realize that baby boomers were not the first generation to engage in premarital sex or to have abortions. According to a report in *U.S. News & World Report*, while 80 percent of today's women and 90 percent of men have engaged in sex before marriage, in the 1920s, that figure was 50 percent of women and 80 percent of men.[10] Those men and women are now the grandparents of baby boomers. One of my clients discovered that her grandmother, a leader in the French Resistance in World War II, had had nine abortions before giving birth to her only child.

In 1912, an estimated 100,000 illegal abortions were performed each year in New York City alone.[11] In 1916, Margaret Sanger opened the country's first birth-control clinic. Sanger was a wealthy activist who eventually founded what would become Planned Parenthood. She worked with immigrant women on the Lower East Side of Manhattan, some who attempted self-induced abortions after bearing several children and others who went to unsafe abortionists who worked in unsanitary conditions. The first day Sanger opened the doors to her birth-control clinic—on Amboy Street in Brooklyn, not far from where I practice—she reported seeing women lined up "halfway to the corner ...shawled, hatless, their red hands clasping the chapped smaller ones of their children. All day long and far into the evening, in ever-increasing numbers."[12]

Despite this obvious cry for help, it wasn't until 1950, when Sanger was seventy-one, that she was able to team up with the seventy-five-year-old millionairess Katherine McCormick to commission a team of scientists to create a safe, inexpensive, and easily swallowed contraceptive. Ten years later, as the baby boomer generation was coming of age, Sanger and McCormick's mission was accomplished when birth-control pills became widely available. Then, in 1973, after years of intense pressure by feminist organizations, the Supreme Court granted women the right to have abortions. By 1984, an estimated 50 to 80 million women worldwide were using the pill.[13] Additionally, an estimated 1.5 million legal abortions are performed annually in the United States.

Peggy, forty-four, an architect who works in St. Paul, Minnesota, came of age at a time when her reproductive life was deeply affected by the pill and by legalized abortion. Raised in Wyoming, Peggy began using oral contraceptives when she left home to attend an out-of-town college. "My parents raised me to believe that I would burn in hell if I had sex outside of marriage. They said an illegitimate child would ruin my life. I was terrified of sex until I heard about the pill. From that point on, I never looked back."

At twenty-four, despite her determination to be different from her mother, Peggy slipped up by forgetting to take birth-control pills and became pregnant. Peggy, like the majority of my clients who experienced pregnancies in their early twenties, had an abortion; she explained it was because the baby's father was not ambitious enough and she had just finished graduate school. She would eventually have two more abortions. According to a national study, 72 percent of women who have had abortions have had only one; 15 percent have had two or more.[14]

Peggy's last abortion occurred a year before her marriage to her husband, Steven, an artist with whom she had been living for five years and has been married to for two. Two years before we began working together, immediately after her wedding, she tried to conceive again but had been unsuccessful. Doctors were unable to offer explanations for her problem in conceiving. During our initial consultation, as Peggy discussed her most recent abortion, she realized that it had allowed time for her and Steven to develop a good relationship, and that they had become best friends. But despite having a sound marriage, Peggy still anguished over her abortions, specifically the one she had had with Steven. Peggy was also concerned about the negative response she would receive if her parents knew. Eighty percent of the women in my practice have kept their abortions a secret from their mothers and only a handful have told their fathers. When I ask women about their reluctance to tell their parents, they usually say they would feel ashamed if their parents knew. "My parents would think I was a slut," one young woman said.

Most women walk away feeling regret, but for those who later experience fertility problems, like Peggy, the shame and guilt is profound. I have found that for those women who feel their abortions were absolutely necessary at the time, it is still important to work through any emotional conflicts surrounding this experience. An important factor in opening yourself to conception—and paving the way for conscious parenting—is addressing any shame and regret a woman feels over an abortion. These feelings can affect every cell in our bodies and can compound reproductive problems. Dr. Robert R. Franklin and Dorothy Brockman caution that unresolved feelings associated with a past abortion can "lie dormant, waiting to reappear as anger, rage, depression....[A woman] often will need therapy to help her examine and resolve her feelings about the issue."[15]

Per my suggestion, Peggy and Steven ultimately did a grief ceremony to mourn the loss of the unborn babies, a ritual that I discuss in detail in chapter 5, "The Healing Journey." In addition to working through her childhood conflicts by engaging in several of the processes I describe throughout this book, Peggy found that holding her grief ceremony created an internalized healing environment. Seven months into our work, she conceived, and she and Steven now have a healthy baby boy.

Like many women of the baby boomer generation, Peggy's dedication to her career as an architect also influenced her decision to have her abortions. Gail Sheehy writes, "In the space of one generation, middle- and upper-middle-class Americans decided to defer childbirth for ten to twenty years. This may be the most radical voluntary alteration of the life cycle of all of them."[16] This massive social change freed up the time and energy of millions of women, allowing them to pursue a fulfilling career.

Adapting to a Male-Dominated Workplace

Women have long worked outside the home as domestics, shopkeepers, secretaries, clerks, and farm and factory workers, as well as in cottage industries, schools, and health care facilities. They have also been the single heads of their own families. Only since the 1970s, however, have a large number of women moved into male-dominated professions. In the 1950s, high-achieving women—who courageously paved the way for the millions of baby boomers who would follow in their footsteps— were often considered eccentrics. Yet by 1980, women were in the workforce in record numbers and delaying motherhood—10.5 percent of first-time births were to women thirty and older. By 1990, 18 percent of first-time births were to women thirty and up. This was in great contrast to the 1950s baby boom, when couples started their families at about age twenty and the birthrate doubled.[17]

The economic conditions of the 1980s made it necessary for both parents to work. "The economy of 1986 was not the economy of the early fifties," writes anthropologist Patricia McBroom. "In the later era, only one in five jobs paid a wage high enough to support a family of four on one salary above the poverty level. Two incomes were needed to maintain a middle-class lifestyle."[18]

The fact that women have had to join the workforce is not necessarily the key problem. Our work culture, which was developed by men and tailored exclusively for them, has not changed fundamentally despite the massive entry of women into the workplace. McBroom believes women often transform themselves emotionally to adapt to male-dominated professions: "When the [business] suit goes on in the morning, it carries with it a set of feelings, attitudes, privileges, and responsibilities that are new to a majority of American women....The suit protects vulnerability and hides the self....Very little shows beyond the mask—the smooth, unruffled rational exterior.[19] In an effort to enjoy the benefits of a career, many women have suppressed their femininity to succeed in the business world, and, like their male counterparts, they identify themselves by their work accomplishments. This development has had decided effects on women's sense of their fertility.

Many women who came of age during and shortly after the 1960s chose to identify more closely with their fathers than their mothers because their fathers presented a better role model for achievement outside of the home. In many traditional homes of the past, fathers were the "power" figures, and in an effort to gain the power that women thought their fathers had, many women also emulated their fathers' behavior and attitudes. Men tend to cover up their neediness and vulnerability by relating to the world from a purely rational level. If you were a woman who looked to your father as a role model, you might have adopted this coping mechanism and further separated yourself from your soft, nurturing side typically associated with the mother.

Among my clients whose husbands earn enough to provide for them both, many women tell me, "I can't imagine giving up my work. It brings me great intellectual satisfaction." But they also talk about the emotional difficulty of working in male-dominated environments. One client told me she learned early on in her professional life that if she wanted to compete with men and be perceived as a leader in her field, she needed to display typical masculine traits (even if she was in physical pain or emotional discomfort, she wouldn't let it show). Her desire to become a mother would have contradicted her carefully constructed male persona. "I have my own business now, but when I did work for a corporation, I knew that the rule for women who wanted to succeed was not to talk about becoming a mother." It should not be surprising, then, that almost two-thirds of executive women are childless. This figure takes into account adults who say they do not want to have children as well as those who do but who haven't started trying yet or who have experienced reproductive problems.[20]

Not all female executives say they want to have children, but those who want to conceive but have fertility problems feel their struggle is compounded when they work in a corporation that discourages motherhood. Hilary, forty-one, a Michigan-based auto designer, found herself in a position of having to fight for her reproductive rights as well as her job. This situation came as a surprise to her, because since her high school days, she had worked hard to establish her reputation as a "no-nonsense woman." A prototypical baby boomer, she earned a master's degree and delayed motherhood until the completion of her five-year multimillion-dollar assignment as a program manager—in which capacity she oversaw a team of engineers working on an innovative design for a line of luxury cars. After Hilary had been paid a huge bonus, she and her husband, Peter, a telephone company manager, stopped using birth control.

During our initial consultation, she and Peter stated that they had been trying unsuccessfully to conceive for two years. She said with a dismissive shrug, "The doctors have tested us extensively. One doctor said I'd never get pregnant. But neither he nor anyone seems to know why I can't conceive." As we explored Hilary's family background, I found that it represented two basic elements common to the baby boomer experience: a domineering father and a dependent mother. Hilary's father, a powerful and influential figure in her family and community, was emotionally punishing, critical, rejecting, and withholding. Hilary pushed herself to excel to win his approval, a common pattern for many women who drive themselves to be outstanding. Hilary viewed her mother as loving but a "poor role model." She said, "After Daddy left Mom, she seemed to crumble. She'd been completely dependent on him in every way. Even with Daddy's support checks, since she didn't have a college education, it was hard for her to get her life together." This view of her mother would later reveal why Hilary was so fearful of ever needing to depend on anyone.

While working for the auto company, Hilary worked hard and

steadily moved up through management ranks. Later, her quest to have a baby would put her in the position of having to, as she put it, "fight harder than any man" to save her job. As soon as word spread in the division that she was trying to conceive, her supervisor stopped giving her choice assignments. At first, Hilary was afraid to confront him about his discriminatory behavior. She had grown up viewing her mother as powerless, and she felt that she was, too. Despite her professional success, her mother's low self-image as "the uneducated housewife" was deeply ingrained in Hilary's psyche.

While her mother had always championed Hilary's academic and professional successes, she had also constantly questioned and second-guessed most of her daughter's decisions. Because Hilary had a deep need to remain close to her mother, she had denied and suppressed just how angry she felt about her mother's undermining behavior. But during a session, she said angrily, "I told my mother that even if I have a child, I plan to continue working. She had the nerve to suggest that I would be an inadequate mother, just because I didn't plan to do things the way she had. It was amazing. I'd never allowed myself to be angry with my mother before, but I was now."

After Hilary's initial confrontation with her mother, she felt her therapeutic work was really working for her. She was able to let down her guard. She called her husband and asked him to come home to comfort her. He was surprised and delighted that she needed him. "I don't think I have ever told anyone 'I need you,'" she admitted. "I never thought anyone would really be there for me, so I haven't allowed myself to feel vulnerable and needy. Peter rushed home to me. When that door flew open, I was so glad to see him."

That evening, in Hilary's willingness to be vulnerable, she and Peter experienced a rare level of intimacy. A few weeks later, Hilary discovered she was pregnant. She felt strongly that our work together had helped her release some of her pent-up rage over her parents' hurtful actions, paving the way for her to conceive. Hilary was beginning to understand that being feminine did not mean being as weak and passive as her mother.

After giving birth to her daughter, she returned to work full-time.

Occasionally, she took her daughter to the office and would nurse her there. She said, "I'm proud of being a woman. Breast-feeding is one more facet of my femininity."

A Healthy View of Femininity

Receptivity is essential to conscious conception. I define receptive as a key state of readiness central to reproduction—not receptivity in the old-fashioned sense of the woman being a warm and cozy receptacle in which the male seed can grow. Receptivity is an emotional and physical state in which our biological creativity rests. This is reflected in the intricately synchronized process leading to the implantation of the fertilized egg in the uterine cavity, and in the endocrine system that jump-starts the reproductive process. Hormones are effective only after they have located the receptor molecules to which their messages are addressed.

Like many women of her generation, Hilary had taken her rejection of traditional role models to the extreme by denying herself any sense of femininity, including the use of her reproductive abilities. In another age, perhaps, the word *femininity* might not have required much analysis. Sylvia Ann Hewlett writes that during the postwar years, the sex act was considered a model for femininity, when a woman was expected to be passive and accepting.[21] Yet that notion of femininity has changed drastically. Today, it is generally recognized that healthy women have a balance of traditionally feminine and masculine characteristics. To succeed professionally, for instance, a woman must be competitive and creative. Whether you became a successful surgeon, CEO, police chief, ballerina, nurse, teacher, truck driver, or mother or father, you need to balance many different parts of yourself.

By integrating our masculine and feminine aspects, we feel empowered. Clarissa Pinkola Estés has written, "While each side of a woman's nature represents a separate entity with different functions and discriminate knowledge, they must, like the brain with its *corpus callosum*, have a knowing or a translation of one another and therefore function as a whole. If a woman hides one side and favors one side too much, she lives a very lopsided life, which does not give her access to her entire power."[22]

Millions of baby boomers took an exponentially larger step away from the feminine represented by mother, home, and body than any group that had preceded them. Thus, little was known about how to support them in sustaining a healthy balance between mother- and father-centered values, between the "inner" and "outer" worlds. Many were left out of touch with one of the most powerful aspects of their being—their receptivity.

An intense and result-oriented focus in life can affect a woman's receptivity. Dr. Northrup observes that many women who have reproductive problems "are working sixty to eighty hours per week, and are exhausted; then they pursue having a child as though they were writing a Ph.D. dissertation. Conceiving a child is a receptive act, not a marathon event that can be programmed into your Day Timer."[23]

One woman whose story illustrates why a state of receptivity is necessary for conception is Hope, who is thirty-nine, the chair of one of Pennsylvania's top engineering schools. Hope's job is her life. As many career-oriented women know too well, her personal life was often appropriated by work-related needs and crises. During one of our sessions, she laughed and said, "I'm the guy who knows how to get things moving. I just happen to be the right-hand man in terms of these computers because I'm so tenacious."

I asked her to take a reading on her biofeedback card, which has a heat-sensitive disk that changes color in response to the temperature of your fingertips, offering feedback on the level of tension being held in your musculature. (See Resources for information about ordering a biofeedback card.) Although Hope said she was happy to work an eighteen-hour day, her card read black, indicating a high level of tension. When the disk is black in response to the coldness of one's fingertips, this reflects constricted blood vessels caused by emotional and muscular tension. More than 60 percent of my clients report being "in the black" most of their waking hours—and generally in the workplace.

I asked Hope how she felt when she referred to herself as "the guy" and "the man." "What would happen to you if you weren't 'the man of the hour,' and told your staff that you needed time to take care of yourself?" She laughed and said, "I know I'm often overly responsible." We began to explore where her need originated to be the "man" of her family. Hope was the youngest in a family of girls. Her father had always longed for a boy, "So I became the tomboy, dressing in jeans and shirts. I thought of my ultrafeminine mother and sisters—who all have children—as weak and ineffectual." As we continued working together, Hope stated that she had a painful relationship with her mother, and that she realized she and her father had been "pals," but that she saw him as lazy and ineffectual. She admitted that although she desperately wanted his approval, she'd rebelled against his life "by accomplishing everything that he didn't. I took it to the extreme. I became the man of the family."

Hope tearfully admitted, "I detest being the man of the family. Men can't conceive and carry babies." She began crying, then added in a whisper, "The outside of me has become so hard, my eggs won't let my husband's sperm in."

Many women who present themselves as highly controlled "masters of the world" are sad and disappointed beneath their elegant attire about their inability to conceive. In describing her eggs as impenetrably hard, Hope had symbolically touched upon the central issue of so many women. As Jungian therapist Linda Leonard believes, women who emphasize only their masculine identity find that it "is often a protective shell...an armor against their own softness, weakness, and vulnerability. The armor protects them positively insofar as it helps them develop professionally and enables them to have a voice in the world of affairs. But insofar as the armor shields them from their own feminine feelings and their soft side, these women tend to become alienated from their own feminine feelings."[24] In rejecting her mother's life, Hope, like many women, had disconnected from the receptive aspects of herself.

During our next session, Hope was amazed to find that her biofeedback card read blue—the highest level of relaxation. She explained that she'd spent the last half hour reading cookbooks and preparing a gourmet meal. While cooking might seem like drudgery for some people, Hope said it reminded her of the good times she'd spent trying out new recipes with her mother, who had died five years earlier. Cooking had put her in touch with her mother's softer, nurturing side, and her own.

The challenge for many women today is to integrate their newly found masculine qualities with a more inclusive sense of femininity. This is a prerequisite for every woman—whether or not she is experiencing fertility problems—to create a new template of nurturance of self and others that replaces the one-sided roles of the past.

Maybe engaging in traditionally feminine activities does not appeal to you. This does not mean that you are not or do not know how to be feminine. There are many other areas in your life in which you may demonstrate your nurturing, caring side—quite possibly without realizing it. For example, many of my female clients who have expressed concern about whether or not they could nurture a baby and be a good mother have shown instinctively maternal qualities toward their animal companions. When I point this out, they are amazed to discover that, indeed, they already have expressed their maternal instincts. Especially for my clients who have not yet had babies, it is through their relationships with their animal companions that they often experience the softer, kinder, and more loving parts of their nature that many say they "never knew were there."

Sondra, thirty-six, a Wall Street investment banker, said repeatedly, "I do not have a nurturing bone in my body." She was on the fast track at work and had married another high-geared banker, Jeff, thirty-nine. They worked long hours, but after two years of marriage, they both felt they were ready to slow down at work and start a family. Sondra came to see me after a year of trying to conceive. She secretly worried that since she had trained herself to be a hard-nosed businesswoman, she had never learned how to be a caregiver, even for herself, which she said was exactly like her mother.

A few months into our work, she told me she had found a sick abandoned kitten in her front garden. Initially, she felt panic-stricken as she scooped up the kitten in her arms, rushed into her house, called the local vet, and canceled her appointments to stay home to care for the kitten. When Jeff arrived home from work, she begged him to let her keep it. He reluctantly agreed and Sondra became the kitten's "mother," nursing her back to health. Her eyes lit up as she told me how the kitten, whom she named Fluffy, had been sleeping on her end of the bed every night since that first night. I asked Sondra what she felt about herself now, doing such a wonderful job caring for an abandoned kitten. She smiled in agreement, feeling that she has within her a whole store of love and nurturing to give to a baby of her own.

No matter what you do in your everyday life, there are many opportunities to demonstrate, and get comfortable with expressing, your nurturing, feminine side. Sondra and Hope are just two examples of people who were afraid that they had lost touch with their femininity but were able to express this side of themselves in other ways.

The Many Faces of Baby Boomers

Although the general issues of workplace pressure and feminine identity apply to all baby boomer women, some women face additional societal pressures that affect their efforts to conceive. Besides the sweeping cultural changes brought about by the sexual revolution and the feminist movement, after the civil rights movement forced open the floodgates of change, many African-American women found their fertility had been affected.

Like their white counterparts, millions of African-American professionals have delayed motherhood until their thirties and forties.[25] Declining fertility rates among the black professional class has long been of concern. The black professional class—which has risen by more than 57 percent since 1973[26]—has a strikingly higher incidence of reproductive problems.[27] In fact, according to the national support group RESOLVE, reproductive problems are one and a half times higher among African Americans than among whites.[28] In 1977, researchers K. G. Mommsen and D. A. Lund found that although there was a 19 percent rate of childlessness among African Americans in general, among whites with doctoral degrees, 16 percent were childless, while that figure for black doctoral holders was 25 percent.[29]

Catherine, a thirty-six-year-old African-American woman who is a vice president of a bank in Pennsylvania, said, "My miscarriages, which have completely baffled my doctors, are more understandable when you think of the tremendous tension involved in being the 'first black this' or 'the only black that.' I've always wondered why African-American women have more fibroids than any other racial group." Fibroids are three to nine times more common among African-American women than among white women.[30]

"From the time I started kindergarten, my mother told me I had to be 'better' than my white classmates," Catherine continued. "I'm still proving to people that I didn't get where I am because of some affirmative-action program, but because I'm good at what I do. I attended a private high school and college, both of which my parents—a lawyer and a businesswoman—paid for. But I have had to explain to coworkers that I didn't grow up in a ghetto, that my family has never been on welfare, and that my father was monogamous and did not desert us. African Americans are the only race in America who are judged by our most helpless members rather than by our most accomplished."

Ellis Cose, the author of *The Rage of a Privileged Class*, writes that as a group, affluent blacks, such as Catherine, are the most disenchanted among all minorities because they once believed hard work and good education would mean full acceptance. Cose cites the results of a 1991 *Los Angeles Times* poll in which an estimated 58 percent of black respondents reported experiencing "job- or education-related prejudice."[31]

The tension that many African Americans experience as a result of feeling discriminated against may be connected to declining fertility rates, according to Dr. Lorraine Bonner, an African-American holistic physician who has long been active in the mind-body field. During a telephone interview, Dr. Bonner explained, "We are often in situations in which we're faced with what I call 'unresolved uncertainties.' Just today one of my white colleagues and I had to call in a medical specialist for a consultation. I checked the list of physicians he'd contacted, and noticed all of them are white. I began suggesting outstanding

African Americans in the field, but my colleague offered a rationale for why each one of these physicians was not quite right."

Dr. Bonner explained that although she's been friends with this physician since their days at Stanford Medical School, she found herself wondering if his choices were motivated by race. She felt that if she asked, he would become defensive and they wouldn't have an honest conversation. "So I just let it go. But my mind-body didn't let it go. The situation had created tension. Although my conscious mind had resolved to forget the incident, my mind-body was in conflict with that decision because I felt betrayed and somewhat endangered—not on the basis of what was happening that moment, but, instead, on a centuries-old history of mistreatment by whites."

Dr. Bonner says an accumulation of these "unresolvable uncertainties" causes black professionals who are learning or working in a predominantly white world to feel a heightened level of tension between themselves and their white colleagues. The neurochemical barrage that is associated with the fight-or-flight responses in all human bodies, which can be triggered by a threat to self-esteem or dignity, translates in the body as contraction of the muscles, an acceleration of the cardiovascular system, and the release of "emergency" hormones throughout the body. How does any of this relate to women's fertility struggles?

Dr. Bonner said that women often stop menstruating when they are in extreme tension-provoking situations—such as when they are competing for medals and substantial monetary awards. She explains, "That's because the mind-body knows that in situations of extreme tension, sex organs are our most expendable parts. The mind-body knows that when times are tough, that is not the time to make a baby. Our mind-body needs to have a minimal level of safety before reproduction can happen."

In breaking away from traditional family structures, baby boomers also paved the way for greater acceptance of alternative life choices. This allowed many people among an estimated gay population of fifteen million to express their sexual preferences. Dr. April Martin—a psychologist, parent, and lesbian who struggled with reproductive complications—recalls that in 1969, "The first gay riot at the Stonewall Inn heralded the birth of militancy in the demand for gay rights...five years [later] the American Psychiatric Association removed homosexuality from its manual of mental diseases."[32]

Today, despite well-publicized vitriolic attacks from conservative religious and political groups, estimates of gays and lesbian families in the United States range as high as eight million adults, raising anywhere from six to fourteen million children.[33] With these changes, damaging stereotypical views of homosexual women being less feminine and gay men less masculine are crumbling. As a reflection of these shifting values, homosexual men and women are feeling a greater sense of freedom to express openly their heartfelt desires to become parents. However, just as we saw with the other social changes discussed earlier in the chapter, while social and cultural mores evolve, our deeply held subconscious beliefs are still colored by our upbringings.

As of this writing, I am not aware of any available statistics on how many lesbian women are struggling with reproductive problems. However, this struggle is illustrated by the story of my clients Alice and Victoria, a couple who eventually brought a very beautiful child, Julian, into this world. Alice, the thirty-six-year-old owner of a travel agency in New Jersey, became involved with her lover Victoria, thirty-two, a high school teacher. They eventually married but had very different ideas about becoming parents. Alice said outright, "I'm not interested in becoming a mother." Victoria, on the other hand, had always deeply longed for children. Before agreeing to get married, Victoria had made Alice promise that they would try to have a baby.

Several months after their commitment ceremony, Alice and Victoria decided that since Alice was the older of the two, she would try to conceive. But Alice's attempts—which included being inseminated with the sperm of a known donor, and having two IVFs—ended in disappointment. Her childhood experiences had been tremendously painful. She had been raised by an extremely abusive mother who flew into rages, hitting her indiscriminately. She was so concerned that she would repeat her mother's behavior that unconsciously she could not allow a pregnancy to occur.

After some time, the couple decided that Victoria would try to conceive, but after two years of various medical fertility treatments, she still had not become pregnant. Believing there might be emotional issues blocking her from conceiving, Victoria decided to work with me as well. Unlike Alice, Victoria described her mother as very nurturing "but too busy raising babies to give me much time." She added, "I have always wanted children. Being in a lesbian relationship has made this more difficult, but it has never changed my desire or confidence that Alice and I could provide a stable, warm, and loving home."

I worked with both of them on what Alice eventually described as "internalized homophobia." In the course of our therapy, Alice finally admitted, "I'm ashamed of being a lesbian." Given society's lingering hostility toward the gay community, her discomfort with her lifestyle was not surprising. Alice's parents regarded homosexuals as "untouchables," and their beliefs were so deeply rooted in herself and in her past that they colored the way she viewed herself. Victoria also struggled to identify and to release her anger at her parents and develop a fuller acceptance of herself. Eventually, she conceived. When their son, Julian, was born, both Alice's and Victoria's families united in celebrating his birth. Alice and Victoria are planning to have another child.

Given the turbulent history and rapid developments of the past century, it is surely not surprising that the generation that broke ranks and forged into uncharted territory by redefining what it means to be a woman is struggling with conception in unprecedented numbers. Some women who are now having problems conceiving feel regretful about having deferred motherhood—as so many women in my practice have expressed. They, and most likely you, could not have made any other decisions than the ones they made. We all make decisions based on the pressing needs of the moment, but needs change. According to Dr. Abraham Maslow's theory of human motivation, once our basic needs for food, shelter, clothing, safety, and security "are fairly well gratified, there will emerge…the need for…love and affection and belongingness." We then begin to "feel keenly, as never before, the absence of" a mate "or children" and "will strive with great interest to achieve this goal."[34] For you, and millions of baby boomer women, that need now is to have a baby. If you are a baby boomer, you may want to reflect on the many ways your generation has been courageous enough to challenge the "natural" order of Western society by choosing to delay having children, by entering the workforce, and by creating a new sense of femininity.

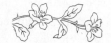

SELF-EXPLORATION

KEEPING A SELF-DISCOVERY JOURNAL

It is vital in the Whole Person Fertility Program[SM] to keep a journal to record your feelings, thoughts, fears, desires, and experiences as well as to complete the exercises throughout this book. So treat yourself. Go out and buy a blank notebook, something beautiful and appealing, to be your special, private Self-Discovery Journal. Don't worry about punctuation, spelling, and grammar. By expressing yourself freely on paper, you can more readily explore early family experiences that you find painful. The primary use of the journal is to record your responses and reactions to what you are reading in this book, especially the reflective questions in the sections marked "For Your Consideration" at the end of each chapter. I recommend, too, that you take a few min-utes every day to record your emotions, using the method I have out-lined in "Charting Your Unexpressed Emotions." One of my clients uses an egg timer when she writes, setting it to ring after ten minutes. Early each weekday morning before the start of her hectic workday, her timer begins clicking and she writes fast and furiously, often dis-covering essential truths about her current life and her childhood.

Therapeutic writing is not about "explicit formulas and abstract exercises," explains writing counselor June Gould. "In the process of writing about my memories in my constant examinations and reexami-nations of the meaning of the events of my life, I had released the powers of my mind with which I could imagine the possibility of changing my own reality. In this process I discovered that I had reclaimed myself."[35]

Testimony to the power of therapeutic writing is my busy office fax machine, which pours out my clients' writings and realizations in a stream of consciousness from all over the world. It is extremely exciting to witness these prolific expressions and emotional breakthroughs in each one's search for their truth.

Charting Your Unexpressed Emotions

In addition to the journal exercises throughout this book, it is helpful to keep a "Daily Diary of Unexpressed Emotions," to heighten your awareness of what you are feeling as you go through your daily interactions, becoming aware of the feelings you are and have been suppressing.

1. You can either make several photocopies of the chart I have provided on page 43 or you can create a similar chart in your journal (perhaps at the back) to fill out every day as you are doing your journal exercises.

2. As needed, use the chart provided to record incidents in which you find yourself "stuffing" your feelings and not giving voice to them. The act of recognition will allow you to begin to release the pressure on your internal organs, blood pressure, heart and pulse rate, and so on. Don't ignore the small indignities of everyday life—their cumulative effect has a greater impact on you than may be apparent. For instance, how do you respond when a relative or coworker calls with yet another request for your help; when your mate forgets to run an errand he promised he would attend to; when your boss challenges you in a meeting; when your mother subtly criticizes your husband or your lifestyle? For every incident you want to record, fill in each column of the chart as indicated.

3. At the end of a week's recording, review your entries to see if there are any patterns. As you look them over, ask yourself these questions: When do I hold back my emotions? With whom? And why? For instance, every time someone asks you for a favor, you may comply immediately. Then later, while doing the favor, you may feel irritated and pressured as you think of all the things you could have been doing for yourself instead of spending your time and energy taking care of others. You might notice that you have a pattern of completing the obligation without ever registering your unspoken displeasure with the person who requested the favor. Your resentment builds. As a result, you may realize that you seem to have a headache or stomachache every time you do something you don't want to do.

4. As you begin to realize the patterns of your responses, you will feel an impetus to start verbalizing your reactions. Take your diary, stand in front of a mirror, and say out loud your responses from the fifth column, "What did you really want to say?" Even if you feel self-conscious at first, practice responding as you would have wanted to. Doing this will make you more self-aware and will serve as an outlet for the feelings you recorded in the third column. You might want to tape-record yourself and play back these responses to remind yourself that you have the right to express your emotional reactions. This process can avoid "stock-piling" your negative feelings, which is so damaging to your body.

5. The net result will be that you become more skillful and effective in stating appropriately what you feel, what you need, and what you want. Later in the book, you will engage in more in-depth emotional-release exercises that will help you express your feelings symbolically to the persons involved. As you more freely express your emotions, you will find that there are fewer incidents to record.

EXAMPLE

DAILY DIARY OF UNEXPRESSED EMOTIONS

TIME OF INCIDENT	WHAT IS HAPPENING? WHERE ARE YOU? WITH WHOM?	WHAT WERE YOU FEELING?	WHAT DID YOU SAY?	WHAT DID YOU REALLY WANT TO SAY?	NOTE ANY PHYSICAL SYMPTOMS
2:00 P.M.	I was in the market and someone stepped on my toes. I was in a lot of pain.	Angry. Annoyed.	The man barely grunted an apology and I said, "That's okay" with a smile on my face so he wouldn't be hurt.	"You clumsy idiot. Why don't you look where you're going?"	Backache and headache

FOR YOUR CONSIDERATION

Have you found that the demands of your professional life keep you at a high-tension, less-receptive state than you might feel is ideal for conception and pregnancy? What are the aspects of yourself with which you would like to reconnect, for example, your feminine side, your nurturing side, your sexual side, and your relaxed side? How do you repress your feelings in the course of a workday? Do you react differently at work than you do at home? Where do you feel the most relaxed? At work? In your home?

Which aspects of yourself do you consider feminine? Which aspects do you consider masculine?

TWO

....

Who Says I Am Too Old?

As we have discussed in the previous chapter, female baby boomers did not capriciously decide to delay childbearing. They were born into a world in which priorities had shifted to meeting essential needs for careers and relationships, and they were convinced that they could be *better* mothers if they first had successful lives of their own. Self-actualization and self-determination are critical components of a self-fulfilling life, and that includes having a baby when the time feels right.

What happens, however, when your doctor says, "You've waited too long—you're too old"?

Dr. Christiane Northrup writes, "A great disservice is done when 'science' undermines the confidence of an entire group of women (everyone over 35) concerning their fertility." She advises, "If you're worried that you won't be able to have children because of your age, please know that this may not be the case at all."[1] She also says that she would prefer to be the physician for a forty-year-old in excellent health who is planning a pregnancy than for a woman of twenty-five who smokes, drinks, and eats junk food to excess.[2]

Another physician with a mind-body focus, Dr. Laurie Green, an OB-GYN practicing in San Francisco, worries that fertility specialists often forget that one of the most important aspects of a doctor's work is giving patients a sense of hope, when there is a reason for them to be hopeful. "Study after study shows that there is a mind-body connection, and that if we convince patients they have no reason to hope, that lack of hope will be reflected in their bodies." She compares a doctor's suggestion to a woman that she is "too old" to have a baby to a doctor telling a women in labor that she's in too much pain and needs drugs—and she labels both as "presumptuous." Dr. Green concludes, "I never say never. I've delivered the baby of a fifty-three-year-old who had undergone a donor egg procedure, and another baby from a patient who'd had her last menstrual period the year before."

I'm concerned that the media's recent inclination to depict women over thirty-five who want babies as "desperate," caught up in a "biological-clock panic," and having "wombs that are too old to work" can damage the sense of self-worth of millions of women. Given that thoughts and beliefs stimulate hormonal secretions and nerve centers throughout our bodies, this litany of dour pronouncements can become biochemical realities in the bodies of women who become convinced they are too old to be mothers.

Participants in a national survey conducted by journalist Gail Sheehy and *Family Circle* magazine reflected similar conflicts. "The dramatic disparity between their actual chronological ages and the inner images of themselves that people in their forties and fifties today carry around in their heads was one of my most consistent findings," wrote Sheehy. "The professional men I have studied just past 50 ... still feel like 40-year-olds. The disparity is even greater for women. While the younger women in the *Family Circle* survey feel only about three years younger than their real ages, on the average, women over 45 feel fully *ten years younger!*"[3] Remember that your emotions affect your body and that your beliefs become your biology. If you feel young enough to have a baby, you probably are.

Fifteen years of clinical experience and theoretical research have convinced me that rather than concentrating on age as a single factor for difficulties in conceiving, it is much more productive to explore painful childhood and adolescent family experiences that create unconscious conflicts affecting pregnancy. But among my hundreds of clients—approximately half of whom are over forty—many have been unfairly and wrongly discouraged by well-meaning friends and relatives, as well as medical professionals, from trying to conceive.

Helen, a landscape artist, sculpts the gardens of some of East Hampton's rich and famous, work that requires her to keep her body in top form, which she does through diet and weight training. When I started working with Helen, she was forty but looked ten years younger. But after five unsuccessful attempts at IVF, Helen no longer felt young, especially after a nurse advised her that if she did get pregnant, her baby would probably have to be delivered by C-section because of her "advanced" age. Helen said, "I felt like I'd been caught trying to pull off that Old Testament miracle, when God gave Abraham and Sarah a baby when she was eighty."

Another client, Shu, a forty-one-year-old Realtor who oversees the relocation efforts of wealthy families from Hong Kong, had a miscarriage after moving from San Francisco to New York. Shu attributed the loss of a pregnancy to the tension involved in her cross-country move. So she was shocked when a New York fertility specialist told her she had miscarried because the quality of her eggs was no longer good because of her age.

In two years of consulting doctors in San Francisco, Shu said age had never been mentioned as a problem. "Since I conceived naturally the first time, I expected to again." But perhaps as a result of the doctor's alarming age pronouncement, Shu began worrying about her periods getting shorter and less heavy. Yet when I asked Shu if she felt too old to be a mother, she said emphatically, "Absolutely not."

Echoing similar sentiments, Kadeesha, the thirty-nine-year-old owner of a Harlem café, grew tired of people discouraging her from her dream. "Some people think it's too late for me to become a mother, but I don't believe that. I lived with my parents until I was thirty because I was putting myself through college and saving for my business. It's as if I didn't become a mature adult until I was thirty." Kadeesha had a healthy baby boy, joining the roster of several of my over-forty clients who have given birth—some after having started menopause.

Good News on the Fertility Front

Dr. Northrup agrees that a woman theoretically can conceive until one year after her last menopausal period,[4] and she points out that women over forty often get pregnant. I have also seen these results with my clients. I've read that a woman's fecundity declines as she ages, but I've also read that in the last twenty years, births to women over forty have increased by 50 percent. In 1991 in the United States, 92,000 women over forty gave birth, and that number is expected to continue rising.[5]

So you see there is definitely a very positive side to becoming pregnant after the age of forty. My clients' experiences are proof that having a baby after forty is a realistic aspiration for many. According to the American College of Obstetricians and Gynecologists, by the year 2000, one in every twelve babies will be born to women thirty-five and older.[6] Journalist Beth Weinhouse points out that "so many women are having healthy pregnancies after thirty-five that many experts gauge risk by health, not age."[7] Although miscarriage rates increase with age, Weinhouse adds, "Most experts agree that for pregnancies that continue past the first trimester, a mother's general health and fitness are more important than how old she happens to be."[8] The women in my practice are typical of most who have delayed childbearing: They tend to be professionals who do not smoke or drink and are in excellent health.

Noting the emphasis on good health among many women who defer motherhood, maternity educator Elizabeth Davis writes, "Increased cardiovascular fitness, nutritional awareness, proficiency in stress management, and attention to lifestyle have forever changed the notion that women over 40 are old.... Age as an indicator of maternal health has generally fallen by the wayside."[9]

And Creighton University sociologist Dr. Shirley Scritchfield suggests that one reason mature women swell the ranks of reproductive statistics is that it's almost impossible to separate out women in their late thirties and early to mid-forties who are trying to get pregnant for the first time—and who might have been able to conceive easily earlier in their lives—from those who would have had fertility problems at any age. Scritchfield agrees that when dealing with fertility problems, a woman's age should be a factor only when she has "unknowingly always been infertile. These are women who, even if they'd tried to get pregnant at age 20 or 27, would have had difficulty despite the best technology."[10]

Among women over forty who are trying to conceive, an estimated 75 percent will turn to doctors for high-tech assistance, and others will have spontaneous pregnancies.[11] Mary Lake Polan, M.D., Ph.D., professor and chair of the Department of Gynecology and Obstetrics at Stanford University School of Medicine, said during a telephone interview that although she cannot explain why, more women who are over forty "spontaneously conceive than the number of women in that age range who try to conceive using IVF."

Numerous women between the ages of forty and forty-eight, convinced that pregnancy was no longer possible for them, stopped using contraceptives and conceived unintentionally. Perhaps that's why women in this age group have abortions for unplanned pregnancies more frequently than any other age group other than that of ages eighteen to twenty-five.[12]

While I want you to maintain foremost in your mind the optimistic statistics that I've just given you, it's important to note one statistic in particular that you've probably heard many times: For a forty-year-old woman, the risk of chromosome abnormality at genetic amniocentesis at sixteen weeks is 5 percent. But I also want you to keep in mind that that also means she has a 95 *percent* chance of having a *perfectly healthy* child.[13]

Remember that when women begin menstruating, we have more than 400,000 ova.[14] As Dr. Northrup asks, "What possible difference can a few years between, say, the ages of 35 and 45 make?"[15] Fortunately, we need just one egg to become pregnant. And since we even have potentially viable eggs at menopause,[16] scientists cannot decisively say when fecundity ends in any individual.[17] Ironically, for the baby boomers who started taking birth control pills during college, according to Monica

Jarrett, Ph.D., a professor of nursing at the University of Washington, "a 40 year old woman who has been taking birth control pills for a good part of her reproductive life—thus inhibiting the release of an egg each month—may actually benefit from having conserved her eggs."[18]

One reason it's difficult to determine when fecundity ends is that women now live an average of thirty years longer than their turn-of-the-century counterparts, and they reach menopause three to four years later, which is bound to have concomitant effects on the reproductive system. The results of a study at the University of Southern California School of Medicine are significant indicators that women over thirty do not have "old" eggs that are less likely to be fertilized. Dr. J. Lane Wong and his associates found that high-quality eggs for donor procedures are just as likely to be found in women ages thirty-one to thirty-nine years old as from ages twenty-one to thirty. "The pregnancy rate was 40 percent among the women who received oocytes from younger women and 41 percent among those who received oocytes from older women. Take-home baby rates were also similar: 26% among those who received oocytes from younger women and 30% among women who received oocytes from older women."[19]

Ironically, despite the "over forty is too old" myth, gonadotropin, known by the brand names Pergonal and Humegon—which are rich in the natural hormones FSH (follicle-stimulating hormone) and LH (luteinizing hormone)—is extracted from the urine of postmenopausal women. Together, donor eggs from mature women and gonadotropin from postmenopausal women are symbolic of a new sisterhood: One woman making it possible for another to become a mother.

The Mind-Body Connection to Assisted Reproductive Technology

The astonishing advances made in recent years in assisted reproductive technology (ART) have been tremendously beneficial to many baby boomer women who have delayed childbearing. In my experience, women and men who have worked through their emotional conflicts and have resolved painful childhood wounds have higher success rates. Hundreds of women have told me of past experiences in which their doctors pronounced their bodies to be in "prime condition" for a successful ART procedure—and of their anguish when the technique did not live up to its promise. I'm convinced that many of these ART failures are connected to the antiquated notion of separating the body from the mind. The "bodies" of these women may have been physically prepared for conception, but emotional conflict may have undermined their chances for a successful pregnancy.

Since its introduction in 1978, in vitro fertilization—one of the most widely used ART procedures—has made possible the birth of forty thousand children.[20] My hope is that the number of successful births will be enhanced due to a growing awareness and application of mind-body techniques—utilizing IVFs or any of the high-tech variations that have proliferated in the last decade.[21] Perhaps the most controversial technique is the egg donor in vitro procedure, in which a couple has another woman's ova fertilized with sperm from the recipient's mate, and the embryo is transferred to the recipient's uterus. While many women feel uncomfortable with the use of a third party's eggs, success rates as high as 35 percent in some clinics are making this an increasingly popular procedure.[22]

Should you elect to utilize one of these procedures, consider scheduling it after you have worked through this book and explored your particular story and emotional issues connected to conception. Many ART procedures are undermined when unresolved emotional conflicts are ignored. One of my clients, Vicky, forty-two, attempted the egg donor procedure with an anonymous Polish donor after her reproductive specialist assured her that she and the donor were excellent matches. But the fertilized eggs did not implant in Vicky's uterus. A week later, as Vicky and I talked over her failed result, she said, "You know, in my Irish-American family, if you were not a family member, you were considered an outsider."

She had already broken the family "code" by marrying a man of a different religion. As Vicky continued to work through her issues by utilizing various processes presented in this book, she realized that she may have unconsciously viewed her husband's sperm and the Polish donor's eggs as "foreigners," and began to work through her issues around her family's deeply ingrained restrictive covenants. Months later, when she tried the donor procedure again, she was successful. Vicky is now three months pregnant and is quite hopeful about becoming a mother. Whatever the circumstances surrounding the procedure you choose, mind-body harmony is crucial.

Although donor procedures between sisters and other blood relatives have the greatest chances for physical compatibility, one of my clients, Joy, found that mind-body consciousness made the difference between whether or not she conceived.

Joy, a forty-three-year-old anchorwoman in Los Angeles, is married to Ricky, forty, a substitute teacher. When Joy began working with me, she and Ricky had been trying unsuccessfully to conceive for three years. Her physician diagnosed her as having "unexplained infertility." Three months into our work, Joy happily announced that her younger sister, Lisa, age thirty-six, a divorcée with a ten-year-old daughter, had volunteered her eggs for a donor procedure.

Joy was deeply moved by her sister's offer. "Lisa and I have a special bond. I helped raise her, since my mother was quite ill after her birth." It was obvious that Joy had become a caretaker at a very young age and had become accustomed to being in charge of their relationship. One of the prerequisites for the egg-donor procedure was for Joy and Lisa to attend a psychological screening process—arranged for by Joy's fertility specialist—to explore the many sensitive issues present in such an arrangement. "The therapist thought we were a good match because my sister and I get along so well," Joy said.

First, an egg donor is administered fertility drugs to bring her menstrual cycles up to the same timing as the recipient, while the recipient receives a series of estrogen and progesterone injections to prepare her endometrium for the embryo's implantation. The donated eggs are then inseminated by the husband's sperm, and then the fertilized eggs are transferred to the recipient's uterus.

After a few sessions, the therapist who worked with the two sisters gave them the green light, in the belief that they fully understood the moral and practical implications of the donorship procedure. Joy also was feeling optimistic as she carefully monitored her medical regimen as well as her sister's in preparation for the procedure. All was going well until Joy began to suspect that Lisa was not sticking to the medication schedule. When Joy confronted Lisa about this, Lisa retorted, "Get off my back!" Joy was shocked by her "sweet little sister's" anger.

As we explored Joy's family experiences, she described her home as a severely emotionally abusive environment, which clearly still had a firm grip on her. The core of our work focused on her "getting real": feeling her experiences and addressing her anger. A strong, successful career woman, she tended to be controlling in her relationships with others. As the date for the egg-donor procedure approached, this need to be frank with herself about her own feelings proved to be crucial in bringing forward problems that could potentially have stood in the way of a successful implant. I suggested to Joy that her sister join us for a session.

Despite the sisters' constant assurances of how close they were, I began to detect in Lisa a strident, angry tone toward her older sister. She had a way of criticizing Joy with a charming smile. As Lisa explained, during their teen years, she and Joy had gone in opposite directions. She said, "Joy was a rebel and I wasn't. I did everything my mother wanted."

I repeatedly urged them to be impeccably honest concerning how they felt about the procedure and about each other, but Joy and Lisa continued to insist that their love for each other was "unconditional" and that each felt "zero" anger toward the other. But finally, when I suggested that Lisa tell Joy how it felt to be bossed around by an older sister, I seemed to have touched a nerve. Struggling to continue smiling, Lisa burst out with this: "You were always in everyone's business, telling everyone what to do and how to do it."

Joy's eyes were wide with surprise. "I didn't know," she said. These words set off a long, emotionally charged dialogue, at the end of which the sisters reconciled and embraced. It was evident that they had experienced a shift in their relationship.

In preparation for the transfer, Joy practiced some visualizations (included in this book) to help attain the desired level of estrogen so that her uterine lining would be ready to receive her sister's embryos. A few weeks later, Joy jubilantly called to say the procedure had been a success and that she was pregnant with twins. Noting my sixteen-hour work days and my love of dancing, Joy laughingly said, "Niravi, I'll be as young as you, seventy-two, when my twins turn thirty." With an emphasis on continuing to grow, rather than growing old, I feel certain that Joy will retain her youthfulness.

Baby Boomers Are Breaking Through Maternal Age Barriers

Age is certainly not viewed as a handicap by my former clients who are now in their mid- to late forties. Speaking proudly of the parent-teacher conferences they attend for their children, these women are often slim, healthy, and at the apex of satisfying adulthood. They have hit their professional stride and have built sound relationships, both of which are beneficial to parenting. These attitudes and life situations are not limited to women in my practice. Their chronological contemporaries share the belief that "older is happier," Gail Sheehy reported. "College-educated, working women over 45 believe they won't hit middle age until 60, and women in their fifties and sixties today do not expect to feel 'old' until they are about 70."[23]

I'm reminded of how much age norms have shifted when I hear clients recall the humiliation they felt concerning their "older" parents, who were about forty-five when my clients were five or six. Their embarrassment is understandable when you consider that up until the last two decades, if a forty-five-year-old woman had a baby, she was often mistaken as her child's grandmother.

Deepak Chopra, M.D., also believes that age is as much a state of mind as it is of the body. "Our cells are constantly eavesdropping on our thoughts and being changed by them....Because the mind influences every cell in the body, human aging is fluid and changeable; it can speed up, slow down, stop for a time, and even reverse itself. Hundreds of research findings from the last three decades have verified that aging is much more dependent on the individual than ever was dreamed of in the past....In reality, the field of human life is open and unbounded. At its deepest level, your body is ageless, your mind timeless."[24]

My view and Chopra's do not deny that we all undergo the aging process and inevitably die. But I do believe that as we age, we have the ability to live every moment to the fullest. We can live younger longer. As a client of mine said, "Mom reached menopause at thirty-five, and from that point on, she thought of herself as old. I'm forty-four, haven't reached menopause yet—and I don't feel old."

Camille, a forty-five-year-old divorced social worker in a Manhattan hospital, is a wonderful example of a woman who broke through maternal age barriers to identify and fulfill her needs and accomplish her dreams. Camille had not used birth control in fifteen years, and she had never become pregnant. She and her new partner, Chip, a forty-eight-year-old attorney, had been trying to conceive for three years. Chip had been tested and found to have good semen quality.

Doctors blamed her fertility problems on her "advanced age." "The first doctor I visited referred to women over thirty-five who are entering motherhood as 'elderly primagravida'; and that's the way he treated me, as if I were elderly." After the physician had read her preliminary data, she said, "The first words out of his mouth were, 'At your age.' Then he showed me graphs and statistics to illustrate the falling rate of ovulation *at my age* and then the rising rate of miscarriage if I was able to conceive *at my age.*"

At the time of our initial consultation, Camille had worked with three fertility specialists and had undergone a hysterosalpingogram—a procedure in which dye is injected into the uterus to aid in the examination of the fallopian tubes. The year before, she'd had successful laser treatment for her endometriosis, and her physician continued to prescribe the fertility drug Clomid to stimulate ovulation. Still, she had not become pregnant.

Camille was heartened to hear of the success I have had with clients who are over forty. I pointed out that although doctors were focusing on her age, she had not used contraceptives since the age of twenty-nine, and that she hadn't become pregnant then, either. Once she was able to take the focus off age, she began exploring the emotional issues blocking her from becoming pregnant. Since our mates "mirror" our past, we looked at her painful romantic dilemma.

Although Camille wanted to have a baby with her current partner, Chip, she was unwilling to marry him because she was still attached emotionally to her ex-husband, Sid, whom she described as self-absorbed. Camille said sadly, "I want to be free of Sid, but it's as if I'm literally addicted to him. He's not good-looking, but he's very smart. He's a sculptor, and I fell in love with him in seconds." Although they were married for twelve years, she says they had no real emotional intimacy, and yet she felt a consuming desire for him.

"When I see him, I think, Now I'm home again. I had orgasms with Sid; that's different from Chip. Sex was great with Sid. But we didn't have sex very often, especially after I told him I wanted a baby."

Chip is Sid's complete opposite, affectionate and expressive. Though her relationship with Chip was healthier and more positive than that with Sid, she didn't feel the same passion for Chip. It was important for Camille to understand why she could not return the affections of someone who loved her, and why she was still yearning for a man who had rejected her.

Camille's attraction for the emotionally unavailable Sid paralleled her relationship with her emotionally distant father. The desire she felt for Sid mirrored the yearning she had felt for her father's attention. Ultimately, as Camille's sense of self-worth increased, she had grown strong enough to divorce Sid, but could not entirely free herself from him emotionally. An essential element in her exploration process was Camille's realization that the two relationships mirrored different aspects of herself: With Sid, she was the wounded child who desperately wanted love and attention from her father; with Chip, she became her own internalized critical mother rejecting him. Her dilemma is a familiar one with many women who have been raised hungering for parental love and nurturance. Exploring the hurtful experiences related to her unmet needs, particularly in relation to her abusive mother, paved the way for Camille to begin healing.

As her forty-fifth birthday approached, Camille realized that grieving over her past had changed her attitude about aging. She recalled that only a year before, she had begun to think of herself as old—just as her mother had considered herself once she reached forty. Camille said, "My work with you has changed my feelings about myself. It's as if I'm waking after sleeping for forty-four years. I've never felt this alive before." Because the Whole Person Fertility Program^SM allows one to release the energy necessary for becoming pregnant—an energy that may have been blocked by long-standing unresolved emotional conflicts—utilizing the exercises and techniques, many clients report feeling younger and more energetic. Camille was beginning to view herself as a powerful fertile woman.

Six months into our work, Camille made an important connection. "Since Sid is my emotional replacement for my father, I felt I had to be loyal to him. I haven't allowed myself to have an orgasm with Chip because it felt like I was betraying Sid as my father." The next time she saw Sid, Camille was amazed to realize she felt nothing for him. She could finally see him as the cold, unavailable, and egotistical person that he had always been. For the first time, she began to feel she was freeing herself from the past. She was elated. As we continued working through her conflicts, the question looming was whether or not she would be able to accept the intimacy and love Chip offered. As Camille continued her inner journey, she realized that anytime Chip acted needy—even if he complained of an occasional backache—he reminded her of her mother. She had been so emotionally needy that there had been no room for Camille's feelings in her childhood home. When she was able to separate her anger at her mother from her feelings for Chip, and accept him as he truly was, she fell deeply in love with him. They were able to develop the deep sexual intimacy so essential for couples struggling to conceive. They set a wedding date.

Soon after, Camille described this dream: "It was two days before my period. I went into labor and gave birth to a beautiful baby, and there was no pain. The baby felt like a girl and had lots of red hair. It was a wonderful dream. Since I'm not pregnant, I assume it's a message about the healthy inner child growing inside of me. If only it were a prophetic dream."

It was. A week later, Camille stepped into my office and sang out, "I'm pregnant! I've been pregnant for three weeks and didn't even know it. It's so hard for me even to imagine it. My life has totally changed. I'll be pregnant for my wedding." We both laughed with joy!

Eight months after her wedding, I looked at a photograph that she'd sent, astonished that anyone had ever considered her old. In the photo, her face, flushed from the rigors of labor, looked youthful and radiant. Encircled in Chip's arms, Camille, forty-five years young, cradled their newborn son, Al.

The "too oldisms" that currently are prevalent in our culture are a smoke screen for much larger family and personal issues that affect your mind and body. Joy's and Camille's stories show how women can work through negative age labels and clear the path for pregnancy by engaging in the Whole Person Fertility Program^{SM}. Whether or not you choose to use medical reproductive technology, you will benefit from exploring your current emotional issues and family history, as both Joy and Camille, as well as many others in my practice, have done, using the techniques described in Part Two.

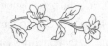

SELF-EXPLORATION

ASSESSING YOUR ATTITUDES TOWARD YOUR BODY

One of the first steps in developing and sustaining sexual intimacy between you and your mate—often affected by the physically invasive nature and the regimen of medical fertility treatments—is developing a better understanding of your attitude toward your body. You might feel upset with your own body—feeling it is betraying you—or alienated from your body at just the time when you need to be most comfortable with yourself. You might also feel irritable and upset with your spouse at a time when intimacy between you is crucial for conception to occur. Many of my clients, male and female, complain about the loss of passion and tenderness between them in the wake of the medical baby-making routine. Undergoing high-tech fertility treatments often masks or exacerbates preexisting problems between a couple. If you are willing to look closely at your inherited sexual attitudes, however, eventually you can free yourself from those that interfere with experiencing yourself as a sensual and sexual person open to seeing how your past issues affect your current efforts to conceive. You will especially want to work at creating a solid foundation of intimacy with your mate that can grow as you face these overwhelming pressures.

Fill out and review the self-assessment checklist on page 60. It will help you sort out attitudes about yourself and your body that stem from your childhood, attitudes and issues that reflect fundamental strengths or problems in your relationship with your mate, and any issues that are the result of the pressures you feel to conceive. This checklist will help you assess the degree of sexual freedom of expression you enjoy—or don't—and how this is tied in with your sexual attitudes, particularly those you inherited from your mother and father. These attitudes all affect your efforts to conceive. As you learn how to connect with the innate wisdom of your body and regain that inner sense of trust in your body that you may have lost, you will free your natural ability to conceive.

1. Make a photocopy of the following pages and then fill out the "Assessing Your Attitudes Toward Your Body and Sexuality" checklist by checking off those descriptions that apply to you. At this point, simply answer from a gut level and go with your instinctive response. There will be instructions on how to analyze your responses later. One of the benefits of this self-guided journey is that you have the freedom to be completely candid in your responses to this exercise.

    As you participate in this exercise, be mindful of how you are feeling. On a page in your journal, list all the descriptive words that apply to you.

ASSESSING YOUR ATTITUDES TOWARD YOUR BODY AND SEXUALITY

A. Feelings, Beliefs, and Behaviors

___ Don't let femininity show

___ Afraid your body isn't good enough

___ Hate being a woman

___ Act childishly to avoid sexuality

___ Feel that you are not a real woman

___ Believe having sex means being taken advantage of

___ Jealous of the opposite sex

___ Jealous of the same sex

___ See sex as a duty to your spouse

___ Make yourself unlovable

___ Fearful of opposite sex

___ Compulsive sexuality

___ Fearful of same sex

___ Sexually overaggressive

___ Feelings of homosexuality

___ Disappointed in women

___ Femme fatale

___ Disappointed in men

___ Stereotypical sex roles

___ Impotent

___ Flaunt body

___ Premature ejaculation

___ Use sex as a reward

___ Frigid

___ Must seduce everybody

___ Emasculated

__ Sadist

__ Embarrassed to talk about sexual issues

__ Masochist

__ Sexually frustrated

__ See everything as sexual

__ Sex is vulgar

__ Tell dirty jokes

__ Don't enjoy sex

__ Exhibitionist

__ Sexual cowardice

__ Sense of self-worth through sexual conquest

__ Pleasure seeker

__ Taught to see people nonsexually

__ Sex is battle for supremacy

__ Don't want full impact of pleasure

__ Sex for friendship

__ Afraid of your body

__ Sex for control

__ Stiff body

__ Sex to avoid conflict

__ Don't like to kiss, touch

__ Sex for security

__ Too tired for sex

B. Admonitions
Have you been told any of the following?

__ Don't masturbate

__ My sexual needs aren't important

__ Don't get pregnant

__ It's all my fault

__ Good girls don't do things like that

__ What will the neighbors think?

__ Mother/Father knows best

__ Don't have orgasms

__ Don't be homosexual

__ Don't talk about sex

__ Don't surpass your parent as a woman

__ Don't feel good

__ Look sexy, but don't put out

__ Keep away from intimate relationships

__ Sex is dirty/disappointing/taboo

__ Taking care of my body isn't important

__ Sex doesn't exist

__ My genitals are dirty

__ Don't have sex unless I'm married

__ I should be ashamed of myself

__ Don't be sexual

__ Don't have desires

__ Don't have children

2. As you look over your responses, what feelings do they evoke?

3. To get further insights into how your parents influenced your sexual attitudes, do the following visualizations. Afterward, we'll return to the checklist and work with it some more.

Close your eyes, take several deep breaths, and visualize your mother. How comfortable does she seem with her body? How does she stand, sit, or carry herself? What physical characteristics do you see she has? What physical habits or movements are characteristically hers? Which of them, if any, do you share? Which do you avoid? How does seeing your mother make you feel? What verbal and nonverbal messages do you receive from your mother concerning your body and sexuality?

When you have finished visualizing your mother, do the same for your father. How comfortable does he seem with his body? How does he stand, sit, or carry himself? What physical characteristics do you see he has? What physical habits or movements are characteristically his? Which of them, if any, do you share? Which do you avoid? How does seeing your father make you feel? What verbal and nonverbal messages do you receive from your father concerning your body and sexuality?

When you have finished visualizing your father, visualize your parents together and note if their bearing changed around each other. When you have completed this visualization, open your eyes.

4. Review your answers to the checklist. Note beside each of your entries an *M* for Mother or *F* for Father (or both) to indicate which of your current beliefs and behaviors were influenced by which parent.

5. As you look down your annotated list, see which of your parents most affected your sexual attitudes, feelings, and behavior. Write your responses to the following questions in your journal, noting again any reactions in your body.
   a. What are the differences/similarities between yourself and your mother? and your father?
   b. How do their attitudes affect the way you view yourself as a woman or as a man? Are these attitudes affecting your sexual life today?

    c. How do you feel toward your parents concerning any problems you may be having as a result of their sexual attitudes?

    d. Do you see any connections to your reproductive issues?

6. As you work through this exercise, strong emotional reactions may arise from reviewing your early-childhood experiences. Stay with these feelings and express them in a way that is comfortable for you: Write in your journal or compose a letter to yourself, your mate, or your parents; discuss your feelings with your mate, a sympathetic friend, or a therapist. Above all, express—do not repress—your feelings. In acknowledging that these feelings do exist, particularly if you have negative attitudes toward sexuality, expressing your concerns openly—particularly to your mate— allows you to heal yourself and your relationship.

Mate or Significant Other

I have found that it can also be beneficial to have your mate respond to this list. This can help you both see where you are in or out of sync with one another sexually. As you continue to explore your issues, you will find that greater intimacy allows you to freely discuss the barriers that get in the way of attaining sexual satisfaction in your relationship.

FOR YOUR CONSIDERATION

Exploring Your Feelings and Perceptions About Age

Mary, the thirty-nine-year-old president of a marketing firm, recalled yearning for the kind of "young mother" her friends had. She vowed she would never be, in her words, "a forty-year-old with gray hair, taking my child to kindergarten." I suggested that she might want to explore whether her memories of her mother as matronly and unhappy were fueling her fears of re-creating that life for a child of her own.

This view of being old goes back many generations. Consider, for example, how, as a child, you viewed your grandparents. How much older were they than your parents? What was the age gap between you and your grandparents? Did they seem young or old to you? What were your mother's and father's ages when you were born? Also, if your mother and father viewed themselves as "older" parents when you were a child, you, too, might want to consider how their views of themselves affected their choices and, ultimately, your life. And if your parents did consider themselves older, how has that image they modeled for you affected your self-image? What are your feelings about age—generally and in terms of conception? Also, consider how your parents regarded aging, particularly your mother: Was she afraid of getting old? Finally, compare your life today with that of your mother and father when they were the age you are now. Are there more differences or more similarities?

Take a few minutes to consider your initial reaction on hearing yourself or your reproductive organs labeled as "infertile," "too old," "inadequate," "incompetent," or any other damaging, negative terms. How does that connect with the way you have been feeling about yourself? Write down all of these feelings in your journal.

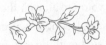

SELF-EXPLORATION

RIDING THE WINGS OF THE BUTTERFLY

This exercise will help you celebrate yourself as a sensual, sexual, fertile being. You can do this exercise as many times as you would like. You and your mate would benefit from doing this visualization prior to having sexual intercourse in order to increase intimacy and relaxation.

Metaphorically, the butterfly is seen as a symbol of your real, true self, emerging from a closed state and opening into the vastness of the universe. This guided visualization can help you connect with this image of yourself. If you would like, tape-record the following and play it back to yourself.

Begin by letting your breath become easy and regular. Your breath is the bridge between your mind and your body. Take a few deep cleansing breaths and feel yourself quieting down.

Lying in a comfortable position, shift your weight so that your head, neck, and spine are in alignment....Gently allow your eyes to close. Place one hand on your belly and simply become aware of the gentle rise and fall of your abdomen as you breathe in and out.

As you bring your awareness to each part of your body, feel your breath arise and fall. There is no reason to make something happen. Become aware of the sensations of pressure, temperature, tingling, pulsing, numbness, or that there are no sensations at all in a particular region of the body....Harmonize your breath with the awareness of your body's inner movement, feeling or sensing as you inhale and exhale that you are breathing out any tension down to your toes, and out of your body, releasing all the tension and toxins from your body.

To deepen your level of relaxation, see yourself counting backward from five to one, in sequence with your breathing. Now inhale, see the number five, and as you exhale, let go of any area of tension in your body. Inhale and see the number four and find yourself going deeper into a state of relaxation. Inhale and see the number three, and go deeper yet. When you see the number two, you will be twice as relaxed as you were when you began. Allow your breathing to be easy and regular, easy and regular. Now see the number one and exhale fully and completely.

See yourself in a beautiful meadow, note the trees, the grass, the birds, the flowers, and their colors. As you look around, see the most beautiful butterflies darting in and out, flitting from one flower to another. Note the very beautiful colors of the butterflies: yellows, purples, white, greens, or whatever colors come to mind. See the butterflies embracing the full spectrum of the wonderful healing energy of colors….As you hear the reflective music that you love, see yourself beginning to sway to its rhythm, as you slowly rise to dance in celebration of your fertility and all that you are experiencing emotionally, physically, sexually, and spiritually. What do you see yourself wearing? What are the colors? How do you feel? Keeping your breathing very open, see the brilliant rays of the sun shining down upon you as you celebrate your body. This is your body that you are owning, enjoying, and celebrating. As you continue dancing in the meadows, there is a sudden shower—and you are very wet, your clothing sticking to your frame. Experience the feeling of having your body's contours exposed. Do you feel comfortable? If not, ask yourself what is going on and how you feel about any discomfort you may be experiencing. What do you think your discomfort is about?

Now as the sun slowly emerges through the clouds, the rain begins to taper off and once again you see yourself dancing in the meadow, allowing the breezes to blow through your hair and your clothing. At some point see a butterfly…a very, very special butterfly. What are its colors? It is a lot larger than the rest, large enough to invite you to hop on board. How are you feeling about accepting this invitation? Do you see yourself hopping onto the butterfly? Or do you feel a resistance? Now, with its glorious-colored wings spread wide, allow the butterfly to take you on a trip into the crystal-clear blue sky.…Just feel your body, your wonderful warm body alive and pulsating with the energy of all of nature around you. And curiously enough, at some point, you can almost begin to feel yourself metamorphose into the butterfly. What would it be like for you to become this exquisitely colored, fragile butterfly, flitting all over the meadow? Note any reaction in your body. Is your mind saying things like, "You cannot be a butterfly," "You can't fly," or "You'll fall and get hurt"? (How many times have you heard expressions such as these as a child when you wanted to be adventuresome—or were you?) Are you allowing yourself to fully enjoy this experience? Release yourself into this wonderful metamorphosis. And breathe … breathe in the fresh air.…Now slowly see yourself coming back to earth as a butterfly, enjoying yourself playing with all the flowers, darting here and there, rising into the air and then coming back down…allowing yourself to fully enjoy this experience. At some point see yourself slowly assuming your original form. How do you feel returning to earth? Now see yourself back in the meadow, dancing in celebration of your momentary life as a butterfly, and in celebration of your sensuality, sexuality, and fertility. Know that in your imagination, as you close your eyes, you can again become your butterfly. In the world of imagination, all is possible. As you begin moving out of the meadow, take a couple of deep breaths, counting from one to five as you slowly bring your consciousness back into the room, opening your eyes, aware and fully exhilarated by your flight.

You might want to write about this experience: what you were feeling as the butterfly and what it meant for you to resume your original form. Does the butterfly have any meaning for you? Any memories? You might want to do a drawing of the butterfly—and note the colors you are using.

PART TWO

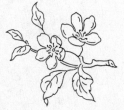

*What Your Childhood
Has to Do with
Your Fertility*

THREE

....

Making the Connection Between Your Emotions and Family and Your Fertility

While we discussed more general issues that are affecting women today in Part One, the crux of the work of the Whole Person Fertility Program[SM] is discovering how your own personal experiences during childhood are now affecting your ability to conceive. When I begin to work with a client, I'm often told, "I had a good childhood. So how can my childhood experiences possibly be connected to my fertility problems?" Clients question and at first even reject the notion that their fertility problems could have anything to do with their families or childhood experiences. Obviously, countless other women have babies without complications, even those who have survived tremendous abuse and trauma. In response to clients' doubts, I indicate, "Children usually aren't aware of how others are treated. When you were two or three years old, you didn't know about comparisons. You lived your life. You were molded by your views of and responses to your experiences, the effects of which you carry with you."

All of us have hurtful unresolved conflicts from childhood that can affect our present-day health and behavior if we don't bring them to consciousness. Think of powerful emotions, such as sorrow or anger, for instance, "as a form of energy which if repressed must come out somewhere,"[1] writes Dr. Leo Madow. Repressing any emotional response can harm any part of your body if it is allowed to remain unrecognized and unresolved. Strong emotions from childhood are like floodwaters pressing against the protective unconscious walls we've erected. The more we force those emotions back, however, the more difficult it is to keep them contained. They leak out into our present-day lives, even at times when we feel we have everything to be happy about. What were some of your painful childhood experiences? Do you see any effect of these experiences in your life now?

Today it is important to realize that your current responses to tension-provoking situations are often related directly to your family conditioning and early-childhood experiences. Yet, when we are feeling angry, sad, anxious, lonely, or even depressed, we find it easier to blame "stress" for our problems rather than name what we are truly feeling. By learning to connect your emotional reactions to your experiences in your past history, you can begin to free yourself from energy blockages that are created when you suppress what you are truly feeling. It is the persistent denial of your feelings that negatively influences your health and well-being and, in the area of reproductivity, can throw off the delicate balance of your hormonal system necessary for conception.

It is equally important to realize that it is your response to a life event, not the event itself, that triggers an emotional reaction.

Most of us feel if we really tell people what we feel, it leaves us too vulnerable. However, when we don't express our true feelings, they remain bottled up inside of us. This will contribute to physical and emotional problems, which in turn influence the onset of physical symptoms that can cause difficulty in conceiving.

I tend to avoid using the word *stress* to describe feelings. I agree with Jane E. Brody, a *New York Times* science editor, who wrote in a 1983 article, that "the traditional concept of 'stress' as a demanding life event is too imprecise to use as a measurement of how 'stress' affects your health. What is distressing to one person may be stimulating to another. Rather, the researchers are finding, it is how a person responds to life events, not the events themselves, that influence susceptibility to disease."[2]

If you already are aware of your childhood conflicts and feel you have dealt with many of your childhood issues through therapy or a self-help program, you may still need to do some conscious releasing of the repressed negative emotions. Energy that remains stored in your body will continue to inhibit your ability to conceive.

"I have to tell you," a client said, "I don't have one single childhood memory that I'd consider harmful or unhappy." You may have the same response. Many of us do have happy childhood memories, but many of us also repress the painful ones, which we have buried deep within for the sake of emotional survival. For example, Diane, a thirty-six-year-old fashion designer, persistently remembered her childhood as idyllic, but during one session, as we explored her resentment of her mother's current dependency on her, she imagined herself talking to her mother, and she sobbed, saying, "I do not want you to depend on me; I want to depend on you." As Diane spoke, she realized she was still feeling the hurt as a five-year-old girl seeing herself coming home from school and finding her mother being carried out of the house on a stretcher. Her mother did not return until six months later. "It is still very painful for me to remember how frightened I was about what would happen to my siblings and me."

Most people believe that it is easier and healthier to forget painful childhood experiences, and your friends and family may urge you to avoid emotionally volatile subjects. However, in your willingness to remember and release your emotional ties to past experiences, you free up energy in your mind-body that will help you heal your particular fertility problem. Recalling painful experiences does not mean you need to dwell on them at the expense of happier childhood memories. Invariably, you will find a profound mix of happiness and sadness. This book will help you to understand and work through your negative experiences to arrive ultimately at a place of self-loving and forgiveness for your parents and others as you move on in your life.

Looking at Specific Emotional Responses as Clues

Can you recall an event that evoked a strong negative reaction and feeling in you? Are there any seemingly everyday situations to which you might be described as overreacting? Your strong reaction may have more to do with a childhood experience than with the actual present-day incident. We generally overreact when someone or something puts us in touch with painful childhood memories and emotions we have buried in our unconscious. For instance, let's say you are in a stable relationship. Your mate shows no sign of leaving you but childhood experiences have left you feeling abandoned—either emotionally or physically—and so you project these feelings onto your mate. You are angry or hurt when he's out of touch with you during the day. Or you might panic if he's late arriving home, or feel wounded during the times when he seems preoccupied and unaffectionate. These conditioned responses are so powerful, they can be projected onto almost anyone you encounter. You may find that even perfect strangers can stir up feelings of rejection—for instance, a bank clerk can ruin the rest of the day for you with a rude remark or dismissive attitude. Emotions are rarely logical, and these feelings of rejection and abandonment are almost always tied to your past.

Out of a similar desire to bury a painful past experience, some people underreact and appear to have a limited range of emotional expression. Underreactive people might say, "I don't feel anything at all," even after a disappointment, such as a failed reproductive procedure. These emotional shutdowns may be a response to having been hurt so deeply in childhood that they have learned to numb themselves to prevent any further emotional pain. Although their current lives may seem full and satisfying, the old sadness, pain, and anger still control their emotions, behavior, and physical health. Many young girls especially are still taught to suppress so-called negative or strong emotions, especially anger, and to react to conflicts or disappointment with a smile. For example, Lisa, an executive secretary, had been encouraged as a child always to be pleasant and sail through difficulties by "wearing a bright smile." Even during our sessions, she initially recalled tremendously painful childhood memories while smiling. Many women do this because they have been taught in childhood that "pretty is as pretty does." These fixed smiles are reminders of the tremendous conflict that exists between our mind and body when we are out of touch with what we truly feel.

Once Lisa realized how she had been masking her true emotions for years, her primary reaction was anger—an emotion she had no idea how to express. Psychologist Harriet Lerner believes daughters learn in their early family experiences to keep a lid on their anger.[3] The message in many childhood homes was that girls are made of "sugar and spice and everything nice," an image that leaves women emotionally split: One part feels intense anger and the other dictates, Be quiet; don't get angry; it's not acceptable. In adulthood, many of these women don't know how to express anger directly and in a constructive manner. "Those of us who are locked into ineffective expressions of anger suffer as deeply as those of us who dare not to get angry at all," cautions Lerner.[4] This conflict about our own emotional state inevitably shows up as an ambivalence toward our own lives and selves.

Ambivalence Toward Conception

Not only are men and women culturally conditioned to present a face of toughness and niceness, respectively; we have also been conditioned to believe that we can have only one set of feelings at a time. If we love something, we are supposed to love it entirely; if we hate it, we must reject it completely. Not surprisingly in such an absolute culture, ambivalence about conception is the most prevalent feeling among my clients—but also the most denied. Dr. Nada Stotland, a psychiatrist who specializes in women's health issues, explains that almost everyone has some unconscious ambivalence about pregnancy, at the very least. Because of the overwhelming responsibilities involved in being a parent, this is quite a natural reaction. She cautions, "If we don't work through our unconscious conflicts about our fertility, we're not recognizing that the brain is part of the body and that our mind and body interact with one another in both directions." At first, it might be difficult for you to bring to mind any ambivalence you may have about pregnancy.

Ambivalence has not been considered by the medical community as an important factor in conception, deeply rooted as it often is in our complex personal emotional and physical family history. When I first ask my clients, "Are there any reasons you might *not* want to become pregnant?" many of them are even amazed I would ask such a question. However, you may be unaware of how a part of you may be saying yes to a pregnancy while another part of you is saying no. Understanding that both your yes and no have been conditioned by the past can help free you to make a conscious decision more in harmony with your own true feelings, and open your mind-body to your inherent fertility.

When I continue to press my clients to examine why they might not want to conceive, they often respond, "Why else would I be here if I didn't want to have a baby?" But as I press on, many say, "You know, now that I think about it…" and they begin to list reasons for not wanting a child. Their primary responses include the following fears: losing control of their lives, repeating their parents' mistakes, losing financial security and personal freedom, experiencing career setbacks, experiencing body changes, and losing closeness with their mates. Many people mistakenly believe that discussing or admitting their negative feelings about having children will somehow prevent them from becoming pregnant, although my experience with my clients proves quite the opposite.

Whether your emotions are up front and in your face or hidden behind a veneer of weariness, boredom, depression, illness, or a bright smile, they filter through every organ of your body. Messages are transmitted between our brain and immune and hormonal systems in the form of biochemicals called neuropeptides, the molecules that are received in all organs of the body. Dr. Elliott Dacher explains that neuropeptides are controlled by certain mental states, including "thoughts, feelings and images of stress, helplessness, depression, anger and hostility."[5] Becoming aware of the emotions you have repressed and how they are affecting your body can open you to the possibility of conception.

The Ephistogram: Mapping Your Family History

To gain insight into your own emotional conditioning, you need to examine the patterns of your family members' emotional lives and physical illnesses and symptoms over as many generations as possible. In doing so, you can tap into a vast reservoir of details about your life— what your parents and grandparents felt about their lives, their attitudes toward menstruation, conception, pregnancy, the birthing process, and parenting, and how this affects our difficulty in either conceiving or holding a pregnancy to term. In 1979, I developed the ephistogram, an adaptation of the genogram, which was created by family therapist Murray Bowen. The ephistogram is an emotional/physical family health history that diagrams complex family patterns that can help you understand what circumstances, over many decades, have caused you to experience reproductive problems. Filling out your ephistogram is a powerful method of creating new pathways for healing, conceiving, and carrying a baby to term.

The ephistogram maps out the interconnections and interdependencies of at least three generations—you and your siblings, your parents, siblings of parents, and grandparents. I often compare the process of creating an ephistogram to becoming master detectives of our lives, slowly and meticulously exploring the clues, plots, subplots, and counterplots in our family histories, the dark corners as well as the light. In your effort to understand your family's generational emotional climate, remember that physical symptoms, particularly reproductive problems, are indicative of a person's emotional state. Pioneering therapist Virginia Satir referred to parents as the "architects" of our families. Their relationships—good and bad—serve as models for our current love relationships and our expectations of intimacy. The way in which our parents related to us shaped our self-image and sense of self-worth.

Whether they divorced, remained together in a harmonious union, or something in between, their attitudes and behaviors and the way in which they handled conflict all can provide significant clues in your quest to bear a child.

One of the benefits of the ephistogram is that it can end the cycle of blaming yourself, your body, or your mate for not becoming pregnant as you become more aware of the emotional issues underlying your conception problems. Many of my clients say, "My body is betraying me." Some women worry that doing this work means pointing a finger of blame at their parents. I can assure you that this work is not about blaming anyone. In this process, you are looking to identify and break through the multigenerational patterns that shaped your parents' lives before such patterns affected you. These patterns no doubt affected and hurt your parents sometimes in different ways than they affected you, but they harmed them nevertheless. As the ephistogram decreases self-blame, it helps you gain a greater understanding of your parents, and ultimately compassion for them.

Exploring Your Family Dynamics
Parental Relationships

The ephistogram can also help us uncover the conscious and unconscious internalized parental messages that govern our adult lives. Bob Hoffman, in his book *Nobody Is to Blame*, describes how we "introject" our parents in the very process of being raised by them, by making their thoughts, attitudes, fears, beliefs, and behaviors our own, or rebelling against them.

When I'm asked how someone can escape from the introjected parent, I'm reminded of a client who once stormed into my office, saying, "I'm finally going to get away from my parents. I'm going to Alaska."

"Then you'd better take along a big trunk," I said.

He said, "No, I'm traveling light."

"The trunk is for the parents you hoped to ditch here in Brooklyn," I explained. "They'll go with you even if you go to the moon, unless you work through your conflicts with them."

Hoffman writes, "Children become like their parents by adopting the traits they see displayed in daily life, and this is not genetic. Children react positively or negatively to the actions of those in charge of their upbringing.... The positive qualities which please and the negative qualities which annoy the parents are both adopted by children."[6] The traits that you internalized as a child may have been either displayed openly by your parents or hidden. For instance, many of my clients insist that their parents were not angry because they never yelled. The truth is that simply because some people do not express their anger does not mean they are not angry. The converse is true as well: If you had a mother or father who openly expressed rage as you grew up, you might have suppressed your feelings of anger for fear of sounding like her or him. Parents who have been openly rageful with their children have had a devastating effect on their development. Everyone has some level of anger. If your parents sublimated their own anger, then you unconsciously will appropriate this same trait as your own coping skill to gain their love and approval. This is how we emotionally internalize our parents. Being like our parents on some unconscious level ensures us against abandonment, for if they are always inside us, we are never without them.

This is a difficult concept for most of us to accept, since we adamantly insist that we are different from our parents. But as one of my clients recently said, "I've just begun to realize that I've spent most of my life trying to be different from my parents. I want to stop resisting them so I can find out who I am." Joan Borysenko, Ph.D., cofounder of the Harvard Mind/Body Clinic, has written, "When I was an adolescent I kept a journal in which I listed all of the awful ways my mother treated me. I vowed I would never do these things to my children. Yet when I had kids, I found myself playing out some of my mother's most destructive patterns."[7] Many people fear that they will repeat their parents' negative patterns. One young woman said, "I'm terrified that I will do to my child exactly what my parents did to me."

I hasten to point out, though, that the real freedom from our negative parental conditioning occurs when we stop denying that we are like them. Rather, asking ourselves how we feel, think, act, and react like our parents is the beginning of our separation and healing process.

When we look at our lives in this way, it is easier to bring to light the multigenerational ambivalence about conception that the ephistogram outlines.

The relationship between a parent and a same-sex child is so profound that disassociating from that parent's life has the most significant emotional implications of all familial relationships. For women, our unconscious need to hold on to the mother is powerful. Mothers are "the school we are born into, a school we are students in, a school we are teachers at, all at the same time and for the rest of our lives," writes Clarissa Pinkola Estés, Ph.D.[8] Mother is our connection to who we are as women. Like an electrical connection, when the wires are pulled apart, we lose power. As we saw in chapter 1, the baby boomers in particular radically pulled apart this connection, more decisively than any other generation before them. However, many women did not realize that by emotionally disconnecting from their mothers, they had abandoned intrinsic aspects of themselves, including their reproductive capacity, because mothers are the ones with whom we have our reproductive organs in common.

Clients are often confused by the notion of being disconnected from their mothers. One client, Fatima, pointed out that she and her mother are good friends, while another client, Alice, said, "I feel alienated from my mother. I can't stand her." On the surface, it would certainly appear that Fatima has remained connected to her mother, while Alice has not. But both women found themselves struggling to conceive. What may not be readily apparent to Fatima is that her relationship with her mother may be fraught with unexpressed internalized conflicts that are affecting her fertility. The ephistogram and other exercises in the Whole Person Fertility Program[SM] teach you how to reconnect with your mother's procreative powers while at the same time remaining separate enough to retain your independence and not get caught up in old patterns of behavior.

While the mother-daughter relationship is key in issues concerning a woman's fertility, the father-daughter relationship has major repercussions on a woman's development as well. Whether or not your father was physically present in your home, your relationship with him as a child affects the way you view your body, governs your acceptance of your sexuality, and contributes to how you perceive and relate to your mate—issues that are crucial to conception and carrying a pregnancy to term.

When girls enter puberty, they are grappling with all the psychological and physiological changes in their bodies at the same time as they are developing an awareness of their sexuality. They also become highly curious about the opposite sex and naturally try to turn to their fathers for guidance at this confusing time. But many fathers have a difficult time relating to their daughters when they enter puberty and begin to look womanly and become interested in boys. Fathers often make one of two mistakes: They either emotionally withdraw or act seductively. Both responses can be highly damaging. When a father emotionally withdraws, he makes his daughter feel emotionally abandoned, which undermines her confidence in her sexuality. Later, in adult life, she will choose men who are aloof and distant. If, on the other hand, the father becomes emotionally or physically invasive, he causes his daughter to be filled with shame, self-loathing, and the sense that men cannot be trusted. Later, she generally will select mates who are also abusive.

Reproductively, both experiences are highly significant. Bodily changes are confusing enough, but if you also sensed that you could not be close to your father or protected by him because of those changes, womanhood can seem threatening. As you examine your relationship with your father throughout your childhood, pay special attention to how your relationship with him changed after you reached puberty and try to discover if your critical attitude toward your own body can be traced to messages your father sent you, consciously or unconsciously.

Healing means identifying how you have internalized your mother's and father's negative voices about sexuality, pregnancy, and parenting, and how that prevents you from seeing yourself as a capable woman and a good mother. If your parents were critical, demanding, and perfectionistic, your introjected parent still might be saying no to you. Your body can interpret this negativity as a no to motherhood. Seeing your parents as they truly are allows you to develop an internal sense of balance in your life and a voice of your own, which will lead to a stronger sense of identity and personal power.

Sibling Relationships

Fundamental to understanding your family dynamics is exploring your sibling relationships. While this may initially seem to be an indirect route to understanding your fertility problems, the bonds we forge with siblings are so primal and enduring that they can shape our lives by determining how we feel about ourselves and others. Just a few words from a sibling can provoke highly charged emotions, such as love, hatred, longing, loyalty, disappointment, envy, rivalry, humiliation, and protectiveness. It should not be surprising that these feelings seem to last throughout our lives. Whether our sisters or brothers are our best friends or whether we pretend they don't exist, our relationships with them can offer valuable insights into long-forgotten memories and experiences that may be affecting us reproductively.

I've included three client sibling stories that revealed crucial information on their ephistograms, which helped them to better understand their reproductive issues. These stories have been written to help you get in touch with your own sibling issues—whether or not you were an only child or one of many. You may want to jot down any reflections that come up for you in your journal. They will prove helpful when constructing the sibling section of your ephistogram.

Despite population declines, 83 percent of us have at least one sibling. There are several variations of sibling configurations—including being an only child, the oldest or youngest among many, the unplanned one, the girl who was "supposed" to be a boy, the child who "replaced" a dead sibling, the "mistake," or those who came into the world several years later than a sister or brother. No matter what sibling configuration applies to your family, you did not necessarily share the same childhood experiences as your siblings. Parents treat each child so differently that it usually seems that each sibling had a different set of parents. Most people find it difficult to understand why their siblings aren't more alike. After all, it is likely that you were raised under the same roof, created from the same gene pool, and that your parents passed on the same attitudes and beliefs. However, research reveals "differences between siblings growing up in the same family that are almost as great as those between unrelated children growing up in separate families," notes researchers Dunn, Plomin, and Nettles.[9] Each child grows up in a unique family as the parents' physical, emotional, and economic circumstances shift.

Family therapist Bob Hoffman explains that "the family system changes as time passes. New parents with only one child are different from the parents they become after a second or third child. As the family changes, the situation facing each new child alters, how much so depending on how much the family itself has changed. On the other hand, even when the programming changes little from one child to the next, children who are close in age do not usually respond to it in the same way."[10] Each child experiences his mother's and father's same basic traits, moods, and admonitions, yet they respond differently because each child is not treated the same. This is a difficult concept to understand, particularly when dealing with the subject of sisters—when one conceives and the other doesn't.

Ronny, age forty-two, asked me, "Why can my sister get pregnant so easily, and not me? If my fertility is connected to my family experiences, why has she conceived and I haven't?" There is no easy answer to this very significant question. Linked by their femaleness, sisters share a unique connection, even when they are studies in contrast. But their relationship may be strained when one sister conceives and another doesn't. Many of my clients speak of the ever-present tension that exists between them and their sisters who have had babies. As Barbara Mathias, the author of *Between Sisters*, writes, "Much is left unsaid between fertile and infertile sisters and their mothers."[11] Mathias believes this unexpressed conflict between sisters is particularly damaging because of the intricacies of the sister bond. "The biological sister relationship affects a woman's psychological development."[12] She says that it "serves as a prototype...for relations with others both inside and outside the family."[13]

Although Ronny and her youngest sibling, Joyce, age thirty-eight, were both ignored by their father and berated by their mother, they responded in very different manners to their childhood wounds. Her sister has four children, while Ronny found that her ability to conceive was affected by painful fibroids—benign tumors that grow in the uterus.

As we searched for possible clues to Ronny's unconscious conflicts concerning reproduction, we began to focus on her caustic relationship with her sister. Ronny assured me that she had an excellent relationship with her parents. "My sister ruined my childhood. I'm nothing like her," Ronny said. She explained that at sixteen, Joyce had "disgraced" the family by having a baby out of wedlock, and eventually she had three more children. Her parents' marriage practically came apart because their father blamed their mother for not controlling Joyce's behavior.

Birth-order theory does provide some explanation for the differences between the behavior of Ronny, the oldest child, who "never caused her parents a minute's worry," and her sister, Joyce, who rebelled against her family's moral code. Dr. Kevin Leman believes, for instance, that parents pressure their firstborns to achieve, and, as a result, children like Ronny often grow up overly compliant and eager to please.[14] Leman adds that middle children receive less parental attention and must learn to negotiate with a younger and an older sibling, which can influence them to become shrewd mediators and people pleasers. As for the youngest children of a family, such as Ronny's sister, Leman notes that although they may be the last of the siblings, in their determination not to be "the least," they are often the family's rebels.[15] Of course, you probably know people who *don't* fit into these neatly categorized labels. In a conversation with me, family therapist Meri Wallace cautions that while birth-order position is an important force in shaping a person's development, it cannot be used to forecast definitively an individual's personality characteristics. "A highly pressured firstborn may in fact become a high achiever or resist his parents' expectations completely and drift through life aimlessly as a perpetual underachiever. However, the child's birth-order position can give important clues about the individual's early emotional experiences."

Evidence suggests that parents often prefer the child who has the same birth-order position. As Ronny's ephistogram revealed, this was certainly the case in her family. Ronny's mother, who was the oldest child, often demonstrated her preference for Ronny. A line of favorite daughters ran back through Ronny's family for three generations, causing misery and bitterness. When Ronny saw this pattern, she began to understand that her sister's rebellious behavior occurred in response to her desperate need for closeness to her parents. She realized that she had been displacing the anger she felt toward her parents onto her sister. This often happens in families. For though we might feel perfectly justified in holding on to sibling enmity, most of us would be hesitant to say, "It's really my father I hate." But denying those feelings concerning our parents will not make those feelings disappear. They endure in our minds and bodies and affect our choices, behavior, health, and reproductive system.

In Ronny's home, her sister had been designated the family's black sheep. Although Ronny's sister appeared to be rebelling, rebellion, as we learned earlier, is often a defense against separating from a parent. Joyce was, in fact, so bound to her mother that she was following in her emotional footsteps by having "too many" children to pursue a career. Their mother had dreamed of studying nursing, until she became pregnant with her first child, and subsequently, she had four more children. Extremely embittered, she beat and humiliated both her daughters. Ronny's father spent a great deal of time with Ronny's three brothers but ignored his daughters.

Ronny began to understand that the same experiences that had led Joyce to act out sexually had also contributed to Ronny's difficulty in conceiving. By not expressing her anger with her parents and by misdirecting it at her sister, she kept her body in an extreme state of tension, which led to the growth of her fibroid tumors. As Ronny saw more clearly the truth of her childhood, she was able to release years of pent-up anger at her parents through exercises and techniques taught later in this book, which are referred to as "emotional-release work." As a consequence of our work, she reconciled with her sister and eventually wrote to Joyce, "I now understand what happened to you, and I'm thankful that I have you back in my life as I'd always hoped to experience." A few months later, she was delighted to discover that she was pregnant.

Looking back over your sibling experiences, both positive and negative, you might be tempted to believe that you would have been better off if you'd been an only child. As noted earlier, your problems with your siblings really have more to do with how your parents shaped your family, however, than with your siblings themselves. This dynamic is exemplified in the lives of only children.

Fertility is also affected by *not* having siblings. In healthy families, only children don't have to worry about parental favoritism or dealing with sibling rivalry. In unhealthy families, however, being an only child can be especially difficult. The child has no siblings with whom to commiserate, no cohorts to offer support or encouragement. I often point out that all only children hold three positions at once: the older, younger, and middle child.

Dr. Leman notes that the unabated parental pressure exerted on only children can leave them "seething with inner rebellion," because their lives have been overly structured. Leman also believes that many only children grow up with a sense of low self-worth, since "their standards have always come from adults and have always been high—a little too high. They have never felt quite good enough."[16]

Diana, a forty-four-year-old buyer for a chain of furniture stores, who was diagnosed as having "unexplained infertility," fits into the classic only-child profile. She was raised by parents who were so emotionally overbearing that they "ruled every moment of my life. I was all they had," Diana said.

From the time she was ten, Diana became obsessed with getting her mother's approval. While she doesn't recall ever having had fun with her mother, her mother monopolized all of Diana's free time. Diana's only major act of rebellion occurred a decade ago when she married a part-time blues musician, of whom her mother fiercely disapproved, although her well-to-do parents never openly criticized him. In her efforts to conceive, Diana had undergone a hysterosalpingogram, a postcoital test, a laparoscopy, and four unsuccessful IVFs. But despite her efforts, Diana revealed, "I'm paralyzed with indecision over whether to become pregnant." On one occasion, when she thought she was pregnant, she'd been so frightened that she'd experienced agonizing abdominal pains. She literally could not stomach the idea of becoming a mother.

Diana's ambivalence was fed by her mother's constant recounting of her own "harrowing" experience of how she gave birth to Diana. Many of my clients tell me how their mothers have recounted horrific blow-by-blow details of their births. Telling these stories is an act of passive aggression toward the daughter. The underlying message in Diana's mother's birth stories was: Look how much I've suffered for you. I deserve complete loyalty and compliance from you, forever.

Diana said, "The way my mother described my birth, I imagined that I'd been ripped from her uterus. It terrified me. I felt if I became pregnant, my baby would also be ripped out of me. After my birth, Mom had severe postpartum depression. All my life, I've been waiting for her to say, 'But it was worth it, Diana. We thank God you were born.' I never heard those words." She began sobbing as she added, "I grew up hearing from my parents about how my birth interrupted my father's duck-hunting trip. He preferred shooting ducks to welcoming me into the world. And he was always telling me how hard it was for my mother, about all the sacrifices she'd made raising me. You'd have thought she had a houseful of kids. When I asked my father if he wanted me to have a baby, he said matter-of-factly, 'If you do, we'll rearrange our finances.' He didn't even say he liked the idea, just that he'd talk to his broker. It's weird to think I want this baby as an act of rebellion—because they don't *really* want it—but also I want it as a bid for their approval. If I had a baby, I'd be saying, 'I'll show you. I can have a college degree, a career, and I'll raise a child and really love her.'"

In expressing these feelings, Diana realized that her parents' lack of enthusiasm about having grandchildren was an outgrowth of their emotional inheritance—as revealed on Diana's ephistogram. As Leman has written, "The key question for any only-born person is this: Why were you an only child?"[17] Diana's ephistogram showed that Diana's mother and her maternal grandmother had been only children; and, surprisingly, Diana's father and his paternal grandfather were only children. "My mother conceived again, years after I was born," Diana said, "but the baby was stillborn. What it boils down to is that my family had one child each generation just to continue the line."

At thirty-one, Diana accidentally became pregnant by a man she had been dating. Viewing the baby as a mistake, Diana had an abortion, a decision she now deeply regrets. Having unconsciously absorbed her family's "one-child limit," her paralyzing indecision about conceiving was connected to her transgenerational family's belief that she does not have a right to a "second" child. Over many months, Diana has continued working to free herself from her parents' attitudes that have negatively affected her life in general and her reproductive life in particular.

As Diana's story reveals, your parents' and even your grandparents' sibling configurations and relationships are relevant to your relationship with your own parents. When looking at your ephistogram, search for patterns in sibling configurations throughout the generations. Look for the age differences among siblings and whether or not those sisters or brothers have children. Often, parents repeat their relationship with a particular sibling by relating to their own children in the same manner. For example, a parent who dearly loved her youngest sister might have had especially tender feelings for her youngest child. And unfortunately, the reverse can be true, as well. For instance, maybe your father hated his older brother and then transferred his unresolved rage and hatred onto his oldest son.

When looking at your family history, you also need to take into account miscarried siblings, both yours and your parents'. Also include any siblings who were put up for adoption, were stillborn, or died in infancy or early childhood. Pay particular attention to the death of a sibling throughout your family history. The death of a child is a traumatic loss for a parent, and as a result, the whole family suffers. In previous generations, childhood deaths were more prevalent because there were fewer cures for childhood diseases and because neonatal technology did not exist. Since so little was understood about emotional needs, parents tended to treat such events as a taboo topic, wiping out that lost child's existence in the family and denying their own grief. If this grief is not recognized and dealt with, however, it goes underground in one generation and can resurface in another. As a result, you might need to do some extra detective work to find out these facts for your ephistogram, because most likely such occurrences haven't been discussed openly. If either your mother or your father is no longer alive, often his or her siblings (your aunts and uncles) can be helpful.

Whether or not you knew your deceased sibling, you more than likely may have internalized your parents' grief. The story of Trudy, a forty-four-year-old marine biologist, exemplifies how long-term grief in a family over the death of a sibling can undermine an individual's fertility. Trudy and her husband, Peter, age fifty-one, a reporter in Newport News, Virginia, began working with me on the recommendation of their medical reproductive specialist. Despite several IVF procedures, Trudy's embryos were not attaching to her uterine wall. During our initial interview, Trudy explained that she had never been pregnant, and she added that she felt burdened by her grief over a sibling she had never met. She said, "Three months before I was born, my three-year-old sister, Sarah, was diagnosed as having a fatal heart disease and died within several weeks." She began to cry, obviously still affected forty-four years later by Sarah's death. Turning to her husband, Trudy said, "Nobody, including you, understands why I still feel so much pain for Sarah. I'm not sure I understand it."

Peter responded, "Sometimes you use your sister's death like a

ghoulish fixation. We could be having a great time, laughing and playing, and then all of a sudden Sarah comes up and you feel sad."

While Trudy's mother was pregnant with Trudy, she had spent
twenty-four hours a day in the hospital, watching Sarah slowly lose her
battle for her life. Trudy had, in utero, absorbed her mother's intense
grief. I asked Trudy if she unconsciously feared that should she conceive, her baby would die. Her eyebrows raised in surprise, Trudy said,
"My mother has always said that she and I were so close because we suffered together. But she contained all her feelings inside. She says my
father had told her not to cry, because she had another baby on the way.
She couldn't fully consider Sarah's loss or even mourn. So she carried
on, making arrangements to bury Sarah, while caring for my older
brother, who was five, and worrying whether something would happen
to me in her womb." Obviously, this created a lot of pressure for Trudy's
mother and Trudy herself, who was severely affected by her grieving
mother.

Looking at Trudy's ephistogram, a key pattern emerged. Both
Trudy's parents' youngest siblings had died: Her mother's one-day-old
sister had been dropped by a midwife; her father's infant brother had
died of illness. It wasn't until two days before our session that Trudy had
learned about this family pattern of sibling deaths. She began to understand the full import of her inheritance of family grief over past losses,
as well as Sarah's death. She said, "As far back as I can remember, I
tried desperately to make my family happy. They always seemed so sad."
As children, she and her siblings never discussed Sarah's death. But
they must have sensed one another's feelings.

At sixteen, when she began dating a twenty-four-year-old man, her
parents insisted that she take birth-control pills. Trudy paused as she
concluded, "Even though I gave in and took the pills, I didn't think I
needed them. I felt I'd have trouble getting pregnant." I asked Trudy if
her early presentiments about her reproductive difficulties might be
connected to her mother. Trudy responded, "It wasn't my mother's fault
that she was pregnant with me when she lost Sarah."

Trudy seemed completely out of touch with her anger at her parents for their lack of attention and nurturing. However, she did recog-

nize the importance of saying good-bye to her deceased sister, Sarah. I proposed that we perform a grief ceremony to let go of Sarah, to open up a new emotional space for pregnancy, encouraging her embryos to attach to her uterine wall. Grief ceremonies can be used to mourn any loss. Suggestions for performing your own personalized grief ceremony can be found in chapter 5.

For Trudy, this ceremony began a healing process for cleansing forty-four years of grief, at last breaking the chain of sorrow that threatened future generations of Trudy's family. Trudy felt a new sense of deserving to live. Although she did not conceive a child, her healing work gave her a sense of closure and wholeness. Constructing her family's ephistogram and working through her unhappiness meant that she would not have to mindlessly repeat generations-old dynamics.

You are never the first person in your family to struggle with a particular problem. Harriet Lerner writes, "All of us inherit the unsolved problems of our past; and whatever we are struggling with has its legacy in the struggles of prior generations."[18] In coming to understand your family history, you can begin separating yourself from your parents' grief, anger, and other repressed emotions.

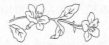

SELF-EXPLORATION

MAPPING YOUR EPHISTOGRAM: AN EMOTIONAL AND PHYSICAL FAMILY HEALTH MAP

As you have learned, each of us is the product of many generations and it is crucial that we develop a detailed history of what has occurred in our families through as many generations as we can trace. For the purposes of this book, I have designed a nonstandard, simplified version of the genogram, created by family therapist Murray Bowen, called the ephistogram, which I developed in 1979 and use in my practice. This ephistogram facilitates the mapping of the family structure, the recording of three generations of family information, and the outlining of patterns of family relationships. In the process of mapping the factual history of our families, we gain perspective on our family members as real people. We see them in the context of the generations that created them and us. We open our family archives to reveal the patterns of thinking and living that inform the way we think and live, which are connected to our problems with conception as well as to all other aspects of our lives.

In the following pages, I provide step-by-step directions for constructing your ephistogram. I recognize that you will be gathering a great deal of information, and some emotionally charged issues will surface. I urge you to consider discussing your feelings with a health-care professional, your mate, a sympathetic family member, or a trusted friend. After constructing your own ephistogram, ask your partner to construct one of his or her own. By examining the larger picture of your lives, you can see if any similar patterns emerge that offer important insights into your relationship.

COLLECTING INFORMATION

You can begin this process by collecting information from relatives: parents, siblings, grandparents, aunts, or uncles. If you grew up in a family in which relatives spoke freely about their childhood memories, it will be easier to obtain the information you need. If you have never known the details of your family story, however, here are some suggestions for how you might go about collecting this sensitive information.

You will be guided in gathering the information you need for your family map by reviewing the lists of questions. In areas for which information is needed, I have found that many of my clients interview as many family members as possible.

As an example, one client's father and mother were only children and in her fact-finding mission the client realized she had never asked them why. Given that she was having difficulty conceiving, this was important information for her to know. When she asked her parents why they were only children, her father said that his birth was so difficult that his mother had her tubes tied. The client's mother revealed that her mother, who was a leading actress, aborted her first pregnancy and after the client's mother's birth, went into a deep depression. For my client, it was painfully clear that children definitely were not wanted on both sides of her family.

One client, Katherine, who was collecting data for her ephistogram, was raised by conservative Christian parents who were strict teetotalers. And yet Katherine had married twice—each time to an alcoholic. When she began researching for her ephistogram, an older sister revealed a carefully guarded family secret that she had known about for years: that both of their parents had been raised in alcoholic families. Katherine was surprised to discover that her parents—known for their rigidity, severity, and bitterness—had been reacting to the shame and humiliation of their own childhoods. With this new information, Katherine realized that she unconsciously had been living out her parents' pasts and reacting against their prejudices by seeking out mates who were her parents' opposites. She was unconsciously reliving her grandparents' pain through her marriages to alcoholics.

Another way to prod memories is to sit down with family members, especially your older relatives, and go through their family photo albums. You could also send letters or make phone calls to relatives and ask for information more directly. Thanks to the enormous popularity of talk shows, many of my clients have found that older relatives are becoming more educated about therapy and more accepting of the need to know about the past and are therefore willing to assist younger family members assemble long-forgotten pieces of family history.

Keep in mind that you are not searching simply for the basic factual information that would be included in a standard biography. While it's merely interesting to know that your maternal grandfather was a farmer, for instance, it is highly significant for your ephistogram that your mother's father lost his farm during the Depression and your mother was born in the midst of economic upheaval. You want information that lets you know the kind of emotional world into which your mother was born, what effect her parents' situation had on her sense of stability, and how, in turn, that affected her mothering of you. Look for ways in which people in your family may have been emotionally affected by their experiences. Start by asking where your family began geographically. Did your father or your mother have to cross an ocean or move from one state to another? If so, did that mean leaving behind family members and other loved ones? Remember, the bottom-line question is always this: How did this affect each of the people involved? Ask questions such as: "What was Uncle Eddy like?" "Why do you think Grandpa would have done that?" "What made Mom so strong?"

Filling Out the Map

Use a large sheet of paper to give yourself ample room to record the diagram and all the nuggets of information — big or small — that you cull from your research. I have created two sample ephistograms for one of my clients, Melanie.

Sample Model A (page 98) is provided as a basic guide for helping you to begin constructing the outline of your ephistogram. Sample Model B (page 99) is provided as a guide to placing your family members on the chart and to then filling out the details of their lives. Your completed ephistogram should look like Sample Model B. You need to create only one ephistogram.

○ FEMALE

□ MALE

⊘ FEMALE DEATH

▨ MALE DEATH

▭ MISCARRIAGE OR STILLBIRTH

In response to the questions presented on the next pages, you undoubtedly will need more space than the chart provides. All such information should be recorded in your journal, particularly your feelings that will be triggered in response to the following questions.

Select whatever information you feel is essential for recording your chart.

Level One: Your Siblings

Any insights about your siblings that you gained from reading "Sibling Relationships" in this chapter can be particularly helpful in this portion of the exercise.

For example, Melanie, thirty-six, has a younger sister, Sandy, thirty-two, who has not been able to conceive. A sibling between them was miscarried soon after Melanie was born. For your ephistogram, mark down you and your siblings (if you have any) by beginning from the bottom of your paper, going from the oldest to youngest—left to right. Be sure to include on your chart any miscarriages, stillbirths, or deaths of siblings in order of their occurrence.

Pertinent facts for your ephistogram include:

a. Names, including nicknames and junior or senior designations; ages; marital status; number of children (indicate if you or any of your siblings were adopted)

b. Educational level/economic status

c. Health status

d. Spiritual or religious attitudes

e. Your relationship to each sibling (Was your brother your best friend? Did you never speak to your sister?)

f. How each sibling views himself (winner? loser?)

g. Siblings' relationships with your parents

h. If there was an untimely death or other absence of a sibling, was someone in the family designated as a "replacement" son or daughter? Was it you?

i. Was there a child born who your parents wished was the opposite sex? Was it you?

j. Was there a mistake/unplanned/unwanted sibling?

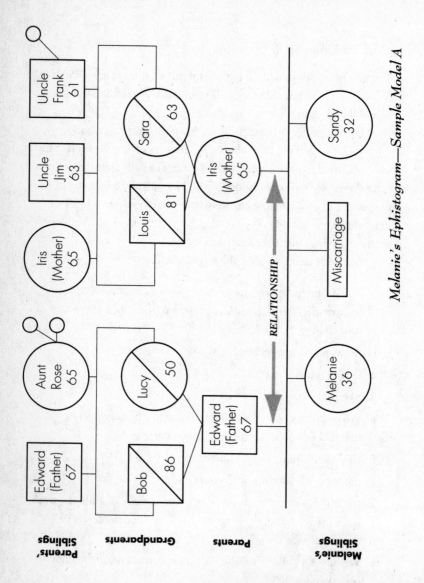

Melanie's Ephistogram—Sample Model A

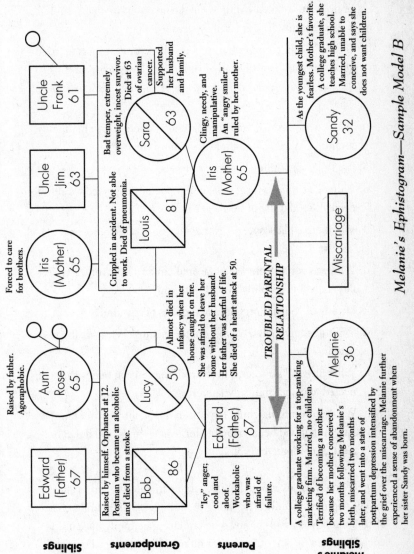

Parents' Siblings

Raised by father. Agoraphobic.

Forced to care for brothers.

Grandparents

Raised by himself. Orphaned at 12. Postman who became an alcoholic and died from a stroke.

Crippled in accident. Not able to work. Died of pneumonia.

Bad temper, extremely overweight, incest survivor. Died at 63 of ovarian cancer. Supported her husband and family.

Almost died in infancy when her house caught on fire. She was afraid to leave her home without her husband. Her father was fearful of life. She died of a heart attack at 50.

Clingy, needy, and manipulative. An "angry smiler" ruled by her mother.

Edward (Father) 67

Aunt Rose 65

Uncle Frank 61

Uncle Jim 63

Iris (Mother) 65

Bob 86

Lucy 50

Louis 81

Sara 63

Iris (Mother) 65

Parents

"Icy" anger; cool and aloof. Workaholic who was afraid of failure.

Edward (Father) 67

TROUBLED PARENTAL RELATIONSHIP

Melanie's Siblings

A college graduate working for a top-ranking marketing firm. Married, no children. Terrified of becoming a mother because her mother conceived two months following Melanie's birth, miscarried two months later, and went into a state of postpartum depression intensified by the grief over the miscarriage. Melanie further experienced a sense of abandonment when her sister Sandy was born.

Melanie 36

Miscarriage

As the youngest child, she is fearless. Mother's favorite. A college graduate, she teaches high school. Married, unable to conceive, and says she does not want children.

Sandy 32

Melanie's Ephistogram—Sample Model B

k. Were any children conceived out of wedlock or put up for adoption? Were you that child? What did an out-of-wedlock child mean in terms of your family system?

l. Is there a split among siblings? (Are all of your brothers married and your sisters not? Do all of your sisters have babies and you do not?) Did any siblings say they did not want children and why?

m. Was anyone named after your mother, father, or another family member? What is the significance of this name?

n. Are there any sibling conflicts or feuds?

o. Is there a sibling who everyone in the family expected would succeed? If so, did she or he succeed?

p. Was there a black sheep—someone who was the rebel or was a "failure"?

q. Who was your parents' least-favored child? The favorite? How did it affect this sibling? What were you?

r. Do any of your siblings have addictions of any kind?

s. Was there any incest? Who were the victims? Who was the perpetrator?

t. What physical symptoms in your siblings do you believe are connected to your family's dynamics?

u. What do you think could have been happening in your family system that had been favorable for your siblings who did conceive as compared to you?

Note: If you were an adopted child, fill out an ephistogram as above for your adoptive family. The thoughts, attitudes, beliefs, and behaviors of your adoptive parents or any other caretaker certainly have influenced your development, no less or no more than those who were raised by their birth parents.

If you have connected with your birth mother, birth father, and any biological relative, fill out an additional ephistogram with as many details as possible about your birth family.

Level Two: Your Parents

Add your parents to your ephistogram (see sample on page 98). If details are not readily available because your parents are deceased, put down whatever information you have:

a. Names and ages (if deceased, put down their ages when they died)

b. Occupations, lifestyle, educational level

c. Current health status (or diagnosis when they died) and medical history; their attitudes toward illness/health and toward the medical system

d. Reproductive history (difficulty conceiving? difficult labor?)

e. When did your parents conceive you? What was going on in their lives at the time?

f. What were the attitudes of each of your parents toward their aging?

g. Indicate if either of your parents was adopted

h. Their relationship with you—or your relationship with them

i. Their relationship with their parents

j. Relationship to each another

k. Spiritual or religious connection

l. Politically conservative or liberal?

m. Was your mother working at the time of your conception? What was her age when you were conceived? Was she torn between her career and duties as a mother?

n. Did your mother wish to have a career and was frustrated by not having one?

o. Was your father torn between his career and his duties as a father?

p. Addictive pattern or other destructive behavior?

Level Three: Your Grandparents

Your grandparents are a decisive influence in your life due to the incredible impact they had in parenting your parents. Knowing as much about them as possible provides valuable information as to what conditioned your parents to behave as they did.

Add your grandparents to your ephistogram. If your parents and grandparents both are deceased, try to locate other relatives who might have information about your grandparents.

As you can see, Melanie's maternal and paternal grandparents are deceased. If you find yourself in similar circumstances, use what information is available. Even if your information is scanty, don't skip this step. Any information can turn out to be surprisingly useful. Use the preceding sample questions for "Level Two: Your Parents" to guide you.

Level Four: Your Parents' Siblings

Use the guide from "Level One: Your Siblings" (page 97) to find out any information available. Above each of your grandparents, use diagonal lines to indicate your parents' siblings in birth order (be sure to include your parents here, too), and represent their children, if there are any, with smaller circles or squares, depending on their sex.

Pay particular attention to similarities between your birth order, your siblings' birth order, and the birth order of your parents and their siblings, since parents often reenact sibling relationships with their children. For instance, do you or a sibling have the same birth-order position of one of your parents' favorite or least-favorite siblings? How might this have affected you? Were you named after any of your mother's or father's siblings? If so, what was the relationship of your parent to the sibling you were named after? How might this have affected you? Did that aunt or uncle have children?

Melanie's parents are both oldest siblings. Melanie's father has a younger sister, Rose, who has two children—a boy and a girl. Melanie's mother has two younger brothers, Jim and Frank. Frank has one son.

ANALYZING THE MAP: FINDING THE CONNECTIONS

Now you're ready to cull significant details from the information you have gathered. Keep in mind that you are looking for family patterns, which may be the block in your family system to conceiving or carrying a pregnancy to term. Look for spoken, unspoken, or hidden messages that tell you about your family—who they are and how your family's history may have provided a script for your life.

QUESTIONS TO SERVE AS A GUIDE IN ANALYZING YOUR EPHISTOGRAM

What family patterns am I acting out?

What were the messages in my family?

What were our family secrets?

Fill in the blanks with as much information as possible on a separate sheet of paper:

I learned early in life that women _____.

I learned early in life that men _____.

My mother and father had _____ in common from their childhoods and that's what attracted them to each other.

It's not surprising that I have trouble conceiving because _____ happened in my family.

_____ swept through my family, hurting everyone in its path.

If it hadn't been for _____, my family might not have survived.

_____ changed the course of my life.

What hurt me the most in my family was _____.

What hurt my mother the most in her family was _____.

What hurt my father the most in his family was _____.

I'm grateful that my family had _____ or I wouldn't be the person I am today.

One of the family dynamics patterns my immediate family has in common with another generation is _____.

I identify the most with _____ (choose a person from a previous generation).

The patterns that appear to tie in to my reproductive difficulties
are _____.

As you look over your completed ephistogram and see the connections you have with other relatives, you may find that your family
history comes alive with new meaning and significance for you.
Melanie's detailed ephistogram Sample Model B (page 99) and my
abridged analysis which follows will give you an idea of how I use this
system in the Whole Person Fertility Program[SM].

ABRIDGED ANALYSIS OF MELANIE'S EPHISTOGRAM

Looking at Melanie's ephistogram dramatically reveals that fear is the
main theme running through her family. Melanie's paternal grandmother, Lucy, narrowly escaped her childhood home when it was
engulfed in flames. As an adult, she was afraid to leave her home without her husband. Melanie's paternal grandfather was orphaned in
childhood and became an alcoholic doing odd jobs. Melanie's father,
internalizing his parents' fears, became a workaholic who was
extremely fearful of failure. Melanie's maternal grandmother, Sara, an
incest survivor, hid her fear of sexual and emotional intimacy by
becoming obese. Sara had to support her husband and children—a
shameful situation for a woman with children in the 1930s—and
raised Melanie's mother to be clingy, manipulative, and fearful.
Despite Melanie's high-ranking marketing job, she admits, "I'm
terrified of being abandoned again by my mother." Melanie told me
she had recurring dreams of dying in childbirth. During her mother's
miscarriage soon after Melanie was born, she felt abandoned by her
mother's deep grief. This heightened Melanie's fear of pregnancy. Her

mother's immediate pregnancy following her miscarriage caused Melanie to feel even more isolated.

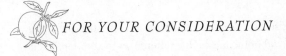 *FOR YOUR CONSIDERATION*

Family Dynamics

What traits do you feel your mother passed on to you? What were her positive and negative characteristics? Did the parenting she received provide her with the love and support she needed to become a person in her own right? Did she pass on to you self-confidence and self-sufficiency, or did she pass on her fears, guilt, and lack of self-acceptance?

What behavior did your father model for you? Did he encourage or discourage you to be like him? What was your relationship with him? How has it affected the way you view yourself as a woman? or as a man? How did his relationship with his father affect the way he fathered you?

Consider what it was like growing up in a household you did not create and living by rules you did not make. What made you frustrated in your household? What rules made you chafe and which did you rebel against?

Consider the ways that your parents taught you to relate to your siblings. Were you encouraged to compete with them? Which of your siblings received the most love and attention? How do you feel as you consider your responses?

What unresolved issues come to mind that may have created and fostered an unhealthy sibling relationship for you? To better understand whether you have been misdirecting your anger toward a sibling that you may actually feel for a parent, consider writing this sibling a letter and explain why you're angry with him or her. When you have finished, ask yourself if you have been repressing similar feelings about one or both of your parents. What role did you play in your family? Were you the family star or the scapegoat, for instance? How did your experience affect you, as well as your relationship with your siblings? How did your role make you different from your siblings? How did it make you similar?

If you have sisters who easily conceived and had successful pregnancies while you did not, consider the differences in your family's circumstances when you were born as compared to when your siblings were. Learn to identify the differences between the way you and your siblings were raised. This will provide you with a fuller understanding of what has contributed to your difficulty in conceiving.

If you are an only child, what were the pluses and minuses of being the one and only? Why do you think your parents had one child? If your parents came from families with only-child generational patterns, how was your life affected by this history? Do you feel your family wanted children? What are your feelings in response?

SELF-EXPLORATION

Now that you have mapped your ephistogram and begun the process of pinpointing the family patterns that may be affecting your fertility, you can begin to link your current attitudes and feelings to specific issues about becoming pregnant. The exercises below will help you make this bridge.

EXPLORING INHERITED AMBIVALENCE ABOUT HAVING A BABY

You may feel you are now ready to conceive—or you may be experiencing fears and conflicting feelings about becoming pregnant. Responses to the following questions can help to clarify conflicts you may be reflecting (knowingly or unknowingly) in your current family life.

This exercise will help you fully explore the reasons for any ambivalence you may have. Take a moment and reflect on why you want and why you may not want a baby. In your journal, draw a line down the middle of the page to make two columns. Mark the first column WHY I DO and write down all your reasons for wanting to become pregnant, no matter how big or small they may be.

When you are done, review your responses and consider the following questions: Which reasons are yours alone? Which are your mate's, your mother's, your father's, your grandparents', your siblings', or your friends'? After you've made your list, recall the reasons your mother gave for wanting children. What were your father's reasons? Your siblings' reasons? Were your parents' reasons for wanting a baby similar to yours or dissimilar? What are your feelings—emotional and physical—when you read your answers to these questions?

Then mark the second column WHY I DON'T and write down all the reasons you do *not* want to have a baby. Initially, you might be resistant to stating any reservations that you may have about having children. As I pointed out in the beginning of the chapter, getting in touch with and expressing negative feelings and conflicts frees up your pent-up emotional energy.

As you review your responses, consider the following questions: Which reasons are yours alone? Which are those of your family members and other loved ones, including mate, mother, father, grandparents, siblings, or friends? As you look over your list, do you recall any statements your mother made about not wanting children? Your father? Your grandparents? Your siblings?

Now compare your answers in both columns. Which are similar? Which are opposites? Putting down these issues on paper and seeing how they fit in the scheme of your entire family will help you put them into perspective and explore what their roots are. Can you see which responses truly reflect your own feelings or those of your mate, or are products of your family conditioning?

Women today generally feel considerably pressured concerning motherhood. You may feel you are ready to conceive—or you may be experiencing fears and conflicting feelings about becoming pregnant. Responses to the following questions can help to clarify conflicts you may be feeling—knowingly or unknowingly—and what these feelings may be reflecting in your current family life. When negative feelings are left unexpressed and unresolved, they hold considerable energy, which can block conception.

If you have any negative feelings about pregnancy, do they reflect any family attitudes toward conception? Explore all the connections possible to further clarify your own feelings.

Take a moment and reflect on why you want and why you may not want a baby. Have your responses been conditioned by family messages? Each woman has her own reasons for wanting and not wanting a baby. Conflicted feelings have an effect physiologically on a woman's reproductive system. Becoming aware of all your feelings is the key. Mixed messages that you are unaware of can throw off your hormonal system's delicate balance that is necessary for conception.

The problem is not being ambivalent but being unaware of conflicted feelings, denying that they exist, or believing that they have nothing to do with the ultimate outcome of your efforts to conceive.

As you look at your responses, what feelings do they evoke?

Your initial response to exploring your family history may be anger, because it is a shock to realize that what you are experiencing in your own life has to some degree been out of your control and predetermined by your family's repetitive patterns of beliefs, attitudes, feelings, and behaviors.

In some respects, this anger is a gift. It is your mind-body's call to arms. Unconscious anger is destructive, but mobilized anger is energy that can transform, heal, and open the way for you to reclaim your reproductive rights. As you may have experienced, women often have difficulty expressing their anger because they were not taught that they had a right to—but it is important that you do so.

To confront this anger, complete the following sentences in your journal as needed:

1. I am angry that _____.
2. When I get angry, I _____.
3. _____ angers me the most about not conceiving.

If your anger is directed toward a particular person, become aware of how your body feels when you refrain from expressing yourself directly. If this anger persists, write a letter in your journal to help discharge your feelings. You do not necessarily need to send the letter, but it is the evidence of the power of your feelings when you express yourself. Visualize a situation in which you expect to interact with the person with whom you are angry and see yourself expressing yourself clearly and calmly and putting a stop to the treatment that angers you.

If your anger is directed toward a situation that is in the past, give yourself permission to release the energy you may be holding in your body from that experience. You might try writing your feelings in your journal or doodling, drawing, or pounding clay or a pillow.

One of my favorites is to sound off loud and clear when I am in my car—safely, of course. I also have advised women and men to take a towel and twist it as you verbally release your feelings—and your gut-level tension. Releasing tension is great for protecting your heart as well.

Congratulate yourself every time you effectively release your anger.

FOUR

The Whole Person Fertility Program^SM in Action

Now that we have examined the broad social forces and personal family dynamics that affect fertility, we are going to take an in-depth view of how the Whole Person Fertility Program^SM works through the story of Alexandra. Although the specific details of your life will undoubtedly differ from those of Alexandra's, her life experience has many characteristics in common with the women I treat in my practice, particularly women of the baby boomer generation. As you read the details of her story, and how her process unfolded, you will have an opportunity to view your life in the larger context presented by the program to help you with your own work.

Alexandra's Story

Alexandra, age thirty-six, an athletic-looking young woman with short blond hair, arrived for our initial consultation dressed in an exquisitely tailored black pantsuit. She had such a commanding personality that within a few minutes of meeting her, I understood how she'd created a successful public-relations firm in Atlanta. Alexandra had flown to New York for our first meeting, and, as I do with several of my out-of-town clients, we conducted many of our follow-up counseling sessions by telephone. Because a client actively works in the program on her own self-discovery and healing as we explore the richness, diversity, and uniqueness of her family history, we are able to build a unique and effective therapeutic relationship via the telephone.

The first step in the Whole Person Fertility Program^SM is to review the client's medical reproductive history. Alexandra, who had never been pregnant, listed the medical procedures she had undergone during three and a half years of high-tech intervention in her quest to conceive: "I have had an endometrial biopsy, a postcoital test, a hysterosalpingogram, a laparoscopy, a hysteroscopy, two intrauterine inseminations, and a cycle of Pergonal."[1] Cyril, her husband of six years, had also been tested and was found to have no physical problems. She said rather angrily, "After all these tests, the only thing the doctors could come up with was a diagnosis of unexplained infertility. That represents forty-three cycles of trying and no pregnancy."

You can probably empathize with Alexandra's intense frustration and disappointment about being left in the dark after trying to achieve a pregnancy through medical reproductive technology. Each year, doctors are unable to offer 160,000 couples—many of whom have made massive investments of hope, time, and money—sufficient explanations about why they haven't conceived or carried a pregnancy to term.[2] Whatever their diagnoses, practically all of my clients have similar complaints.

As a complementary program to medical fertility treatments, the Whole Person Fertility Program^SM can enhance the effectiveness of medical reproductive interventions. While a number of fertility specialists refer clients to me, my process is highly effective whether or not a person is undergoing medical treatments. Alexandra is one of several of my clients who discontinued her medical intervention during the nine months that we worked together.

I had Alexandra fill out a lifestyle profile. Alexandra's profile provided key information about her current life issues and an inkling of her past history that might have been affecting her reproductive life.

Alexandra had written in her profile, "I experience a great deal of nervousness and anxiety, and I lose my temper when things don't go the way I expect them to or think they should." Given that Alexandra is a successful businesswoman accustomed to being in control, it was easy to understand just how tense and angry she felt about not conceiving. Alexandra had also noted in her profile that she has close and supportive relationships with women friends and her family. She also has a good relationship with her husband, Cyril, age thirty-eight, who manages a chain of luxury hotels. "We have a playful relationship and pet names for each other," Alexandra said. "I feel completely natural and at home around him. He very much wants to have children, too, and feels blue when he sees pregnant women." Together for a decade and married for six of those years, Alexandra said they have sex about three times a week.

Alexandra explained that she wanted to have a baby "because Cyril and I have so much love to give. I think I would be a good mother and I know he would be a gentle, loving father. I want to feel a new life growing inside me, to nurse my baby at my breasts, to see the wonder and love in my child's eyes, and to have someone love me, trust me, and need me unconditionally." I was moved by her responses, and since she had no physical problems to prevent her from becoming pregnant, I was determined to help her uncover what was keeping her from realizing her dream. So we went back to explore her childhood in an attempt to discover why she might *not* want to conceive.

At first, Alexandra said she felt no reluctance about becoming pregnant, but later she admitted that she did have ambivalent feelings. When I asked her, "What did you hear or experience about pregnancy or childbirth when you were growing up?" she recalled visiting a farm when she was twelve. This is a crucial time in a girl's life, when her body undergoes major changes she may not understand, and when she is apt to be acutely sensitive to rejection and fearful of being physically imperfect.

"I remember standing in a bedroom window of the farmhouse, where I could look out onto an open airy space with limitless possibilities, but my eyes would always be drawn to the yard below. I was so repulsed by the sight of the sow rooting right through the mud, a trail of piglets squealing behind her. She seemed to be trying to wean them, but they would always catch up and latch on to her swollen teats. She both fascinated and nauseated me. She was everything I didn't want to be—fat, ugly, and existing only to serve the needs of others."

Ironically, though repulsed by the pig and her suckling brood, Alexandra said she also remembered the sight as being erotic. "I felt the same way when I watched the family cow being milked, or a young mother from a nearby household nurse her baby. On some deep level, I, too, wanted to be a nurturing, comforting mother with breasts full of milk for her baby."

Despite Alexandra's cool, professional facade, I sensed it was actually she who longed to be the one receiving the nurturing. Clients who speak of wanting to have a baby to whom they can give unconditional love are often young women or men who never received this kind of love and devotion in their own childhoods. Alexandra said that for many years she had repressed the urge to be nurturing and motherly. "Taking care of babies would have taken attention away from me. I needed attention. Caring for babies was for fat, dumpy girls with no brains," she said. The depth of her conflict concerning motherhood was beginning to reveal itself, particularly as she disclosed her struggle with anorexia during her junior high school years.

"I felt if I could be thin, I could be happy. I ate practically nothing. Through such control, I would prevent my body from becoming fat, vulnerable, and feminine." As a girl, Alexandra had equated being feminine as something her mother looked down upon. She related that her mother, Anne, was "a very bright, strong-willed woman, who was frustrated that she could not develop professionally during the years when I was a child." Alexandra's story touches upon the core dilemma for so many women. They feel starved for the attention and affection they did not receive in childhood; as a result, they become contemptuous of motherhood on a deep level. At the same time, they are unconsciously fearful that if they admit this, they will denigrate or betray their mothers. This dilemma had left Alexandra filled with guilt about her negative images of motherhood. We began mapping her generational family history to understand what had left her so in need of attention and nurturance. (Please see the outline of Alexandra's Ephistogram on the facing page as well as step-by-step directions for composing your own ephistogram, in the previous chapter.) Alexandra and I sifted through her history, searching for critical clues as to why she was having difficulty conceiving. Her responses to my questions began to fill out the larger picture of her life. Her ephistogram is outlined below. As the events of Alexandra's life were revealed in the ephistogram, I learned that her parents are highly regarded theologians who have been married for more than four decades, and that Alexandra's mother, Anne, had been reluctant to become pregnant. As Anne's childhood history unfolded, her reluctance proved understandable.

Alexandra's Family History

Although many of the details of Alexandra's maternal grandparents were lost to time, she did recall hearing that both had become orphans early in their childhoods. Years later, at separate times, they had emigrated from Spain to the United States. Alexandra's mother, Anne, was among the first generation in her family to be born in the United States. "My mother's birth was considered no big deal," said Alexandra, "but the births of her two younger brothers were heralded, especially my grandmother's first son, Raul, who was doted upon." Five-year-old Anne stood on the sidelines, watching as her parents and extended family celebrated Raul's first birthday. Alexandra recalled her mother saying that Raul received a hand-carved toy sailboat that year but that her birthdays were always forgotten.

Anne's father, who was referred to as Mr. Alejandro (for whom Alexandra was named), was sickly. Anne's mother, Constanza, had to give him constant care. That left Anne, at ten, to be the substitute full-time mother for her two younger brothers. Mr. Alejandro died at thirty-nine of a heart attack, when Anne was sixteen. Years later, Constanza

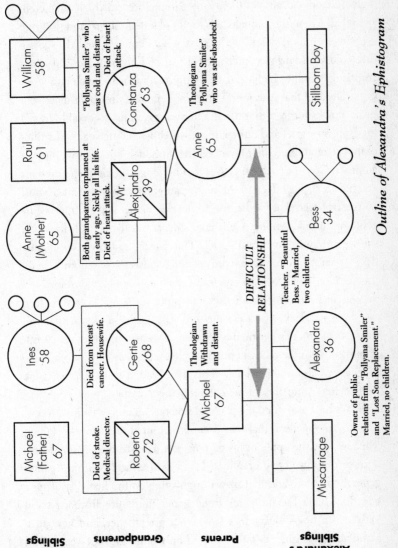

Outline of Alexandra's Ephistogram

also would die from a heart attack. Both Anne's parents were desperately unhappy because of their early parental losses, which were compounded when they emigrated to the United States and lost the emotional support system of their extended family. Given Mr. Alejandro's and Constanza's earlier lives of fear and abandonment, it is not surprising that they had created a highly anxious, fear-driven family.

The fact that Alexandra's maternal grandparents both died from heart attacks suggests that her mother was given no acceptable model for expressing grief and unhappiness, which wasn't unusual for families of that generation. Rather than "getting it off their chests," stoicism was admired. Current research proves that holding in such deep emotions can have a strong effect on the body, particularly on the heart. It must be remembered that the heart is a muscle, and as such, is affected by acute or chronic tension. Constanza's heart was like a vault in which she locked away her private grief. This family trait fits a personality style—seen on Alexandra's ephistogram—passed down from Grandmother Constanza to Anne and to Alexandra. Although Constanza was depressed, she taught Anne always to put on a happy Pollyanna face and hide her feelings—a curious mix of anger and charm that still marked Alexandra's personality. Anne's dazzling smile hid her resentments from childhood, which negatively shaped her view of marriage, pregnancy, and motherhood. This background gave me valuable insights into Anne's resentment about being a mother.

We next examined the paternal side of Alexandra's family. In contrast to the neglect that her mother endured, Alexandra's father, Michael, was the apple of his parents' eye. He was the treasured firstborn son in a well-to-do family that also had emigrated from Spain a generation before and that placed high value on the firstborn being a boy. In Michael's family for three generations, the firstborn child had been a boy—Alexandra's father, her grandfather, and her great-grandfather. Alexandra's father was an only child for nine years, until his sister, Inez, was born.

Michael's parents prized an orderly household, however, and viewed children as necessary disturbances, which explains the protracted delay between Michael's and Inez's births. Even today, nine years would be considered a long wait between children. In the 1930s, it was highly unusual. The need for a quiet house, without the noise and disruption of small children, proved significant in understanding Michael's ambivalent attitude toward Alexandra, which she absorbed.

"My mother told me she married Daddy to please her mother," Alexandra said. "His family was wealthy and my mother's family was poor. It was a tension-filled marriage at the outset." Anne, who longed to have a career, did not complete her Ph.D. in theology until the early seventies because of family and societal pressures that she bear a child. Anne and Michael's first attempt to start a family ended in a miscarriage, and Alexandra was not conceived for another six years—an unusually long wait for a couple in the fifties.

Anne told everyone she was delighted to be pregnant with Alexandra, but her body told another story: She contracted pneumonia. Alexandra said, "They were in Madrid for my father's postdoctoral work. The doctors said I would surely die, and that she, too, might not pull through. They told her she should abort me, but she refused, and fought for my life and hers." On the one hand, Anne loved her unborn child enough to risk her own life; on the other, her illness indicated just how conflicted she was. Anne's pneumonia was a manifestation of her despair. "Lungs are the center of our desires and yearnings to experience more of life," writes Serge King in *Imagineering for Health*.[3] Rather than being joy-filled while pregnant, Alexandra's mother must have felt she was back where she'd left off with her brothers—expected to put her ambitions on hold so she could take care of someone else's needs.

Babies in utero feel vibrationally—through their mother's musculature and body rhythms—the physiological effects of any long-term anxiety, tension, and nervousness. Alexandra's earliest unconscious memories can be traced back to her life in utero. Much of what a pregnant woman thinks, feels, says, and hopes influences her unborn child. "Chronic anxiety or a wrenching ambivalence about motherhood can leave a deep scar on an unborn child's personality,"[4] writes Dr. Thomas Verny, author of *The Secret Life of the Unborn Child*. While an adult learns to deflect difficult experiences, the unborn child cannot. Since a child learns to interpret on a primitive level his mother's emotions, what a woman feels and thinks about her child makes a significant impact on his personality. Dr. Verny writes, "Her thoughts—her love or rejection, or ambivalence—begin defining and shaping his emotional life."[5]

Adding to Alexandra's distressing life in utero was her father's lack of interest in his wife's pregnancy. "How a man feels about his wife and unborn child is one of the single most important factors in determining the success of a pregnancy," writes Dr. Verny.[6] Alexandra's father was often so preoccupied with his work that her mother said when she was pregnant, she felt he would be worried that a child would interfere with his schedule. As we explored further, it was evident that Alexandra's parents' marriage and Alexandra's dismal life in utero set the stage for the way in which her reproductive life would be affected.

By breaking the tradition of firstborn sons in Michael's family, Alexandra felt she must have been a disappointment to her parents. Three years after Alexandra was born, Anne had another daughter, Bess. Two years after Bess's birth, Alexandra's mother became pregnant again. Alexandra vividly recalled her mother telling her about this pregnancy. "She had been helping my father prepare his lectures for translation and he kept pushing her to finish, goading her to keep working." Alexandra said her mother was exhausted, and after six months, the baby was stillborn. It was a boy. "He would have been named after my father," she said. From this experience, Alexandra became convinced that men wield the power in the family, and that women cannot be strong as well as feminine. "I felt my father devalued the nurturing aspect of a woman and felt that taking care of babies was what stupid people do."

The tragedy of the stillborn son widened the division in her family. By the time Alexandra was four years old, she and her father were aligned on one side, and Bess and her mother on the other. The split occurred primarily because her mother focused her anger on Alexandra—anger that was as old as Anne's childhood and as current as her marriage. Alexandra, like her mother, was a firstborn girl, so Anne saw her own unresolved conflicts from the past and her deferred hopes and dreams in Alexandra, and Alexandra was named for the father who had abandoned Anne by his illness and early death. Finally, Alexandra bore a striking resemblance to Michael. "When my mother got angry with me, she would say I was thoughtless and selfish like my father, as well as stubborn, angry, and impatient." Stung by her mother's rejection, Alexandra gravitated toward her father, who offered some warmth and approval. For Michael, Alexandra became a replacement for his still-born son. Alexandra said in an icy voice, "I don't know when it happened, but at some point, I found I was more comfortable dressed like a tomboy."

Anne and Michael's conflicted feelings about their first child were reflected in how they treated her. On the one hand, Alexandra was catered to as the oldest child and given gala birthday celebrations, but on the other hand, Alexandra said, "I can still hear my mother saying, 'No, no. no.' I'm told that my first words were 'No, Alexandra, don't.' Evidently, I was mimicking my mother, who often indicated I wasn't doing things the right way—her way. It made me feel I wasn't good enough. I remember feeling so sad. What had I done wrong?"

Alexandra recalled having nightmares about her mother rejecting her, and she says that in early photographs she was always pictured clutching a stuffed animal. "I remember holding on to my teddy bear so I could feel some tenderness and affection."

Life was different for Bess. Alexandra's mother forged an alliance with her, giving her the sense that motherhood was something to look forward to. You may recall my saying earlier that siblings do not actually share the same parents. Life had also changed for Alexandra's parents by the time Bess came along. Bess was conceived and born after the family had moved back to the States, where Michael had accepted a teaching post in Atlanta. It was a time when her parents were experiencing fewer pressures in their marriage, and Bess happened to resemble Anne. Her parents called her "Beautiful Bess."

When parents use these kinds of nicknames for siblings—indicating that one is "good" and the other "bad" or less desirable—they can severely damage each child and the sibling relationship. Alexandra measured herself according to Bess, and she found herself lacking. She lamented, "Unlike my sister, I was not feminine, not nurturing, not caring. Bess was demure and feminine. She was the girl. I was the boy." On some level, Alexandra knew which role she had been assigned in her family, that of the son who never was.

Alexandra reached out to her father by taking on the role of his lost son. She is intellectual, strong, and competitive—all marvelous attributes in a man or a woman. But from her confused logic as a child, all of those traits meant she also couldn't be womanly. Two months into our work, Alexandra talked about her earliest responses to her mother's rejection. "Deep inside, I felt myself closing. It wasn't muscles tensing. It was much more vague. When I was a child, as far back as four or five, I didn't want to grow into a woman, to develop breasts or have babies. When I got older, I didn't even like my little sister to rest her head in my lap when we sat in the backseat during long car trips."

Alexandra's rejection of herself as a woman did not simply exist in her mind. These emotions permeated every cell of her body. The dramatic differences between Alexandra's childhood experiences and those of her sister, Bess, affected the choices they made about their adult lives. By the time Alexandra had completed graduate school, her sister, who had married early, had her first child after waiting several years, following in her mother's footsteps. Alexandra followed in her father's footsteps and made her life extremely different from her mother's.

Alexandra said, "Bess has a wonderful son and daughter. Each time, she conceived right away, even though she had menstrual irregularities." Alexandra's struggle to conceive, given the fact that her sister had easily become pregnant, created enmity between them.

As Alexandra and I continued our exploration, I asked her to draw sketches of her immediate family. She drew a picture of herself and her sister, Bess, merged into one body but with their heads tilted in opposite directions. The drawings literally reflected that their lives had moved in opposite directions. Alexandra had written, "Little Mother" under the picture of Bess, who is both a mother and teaches preschool. I noted that although Alexandra is the older of the two, Alexandra drew Bess first and herself second—out of sibling order—which suggests an unconscious belief that Bess has higher status in their family.

When we did her photoanalysis (detailed in the next chapter) by looking over her family snapshots, Alexandra remarked, "I really do look isolated." She gazed at a snapshot of her family standing behind a heavily laden Christmas table. Cyril's arms were wrapped around Alexandra, who stood separately from the group that included her mother, father, Bess, and Bess's husband and children. Even with her husband by her side, Alexandra looked sad and alone.

Alexandra's Breakthrough

Several weeks into therapy, Alexandra recounted a painful story that illustrated how she felt emotionally and physically abandoned by her mother. "Mom had said she had to run an errand. My father was out of town and she'd forgotten to put gas in our old blue Dodge. She said she was going to leave me and Bess alone for just a few minutes. I was scared to death. Bess was only three years old. We sat there, the two of us huddled on the front steps, leading to the upstairs, and it seemed like an eternity. I was very scared, very worried. Would she ever come back to us? Twenty minutes later, when she returned, I just heaved a sigh of relief."

When I asked Alexandra how she felt about this experience, she agreed that by almost any standard, six- and three-year-old children are too young to be left alone in a house. This memory signaled the beginning of her recall of additional painful experiences. I encouraged her to use several techniques for emotional release, such as pillow talk (detailed in the next chapter), to confront her feelings of childhood abandonment.

One day when I called Alexandra for our phone session, she was weeping bitterly about an experience at a seminar for women entrepreneurs that had been led by an older woman, whom she described as cold and unloving. During the weekend, this woman called upon other women to speak, yet she consistently ignored Alexandra's attempts to contribute. This inattention was particularly hurtful to Alexandra, since so much of her self-esteem was based on being recognized for making intellectual contributions. Coincidentally, the seminar leader's name was Anne, the same name as Alexandra's mother's. Alexandra was shocked by the degree of her own reaction. She sobbed uncontrollably as she slowly began to admit, "I know this actually has to do with unresolved business about my mother."

She couldn't have been more accurate. The encounter had reawakened the deep-seated unresolved pain Alexandra had experienced in childhood. The workshop leader had ignored her just as her mother had. Alexandra could not deny or suppress her feelings any longer as she had done repeatedly during her life. Our work together had left her vulnerable and she was beginning to feel the full weight of the pain she had buried—the pain of rejection.

After about eight months of working together, Alexandra speculated, "Maybe I haven't been able to conceive because I'm afraid to do to a child what my mother did to me. At first, this idea struck me as absurd. What terrible thing had my mother done to me?...There was nothing I could think of."

For me, it was ironic to hear Alexandra say this, when she had cited chapter and verse her experiences of feeling rejected and neglected. It was apparent to me that it was very difficult for Alexandra, even after many intensive months of working together, to allow herself to accept what had actually happened.

As she continued talking in this vein, however, I realized she had had a major breakthrough. I was terribly excited as she said, "The more I think about this as a possibility, the more it seems to make sense. There had been a lot of anger that I was housing and not giving voice to. Maybe this is what I've been afraid of. Maybe the fear is buried so deep, I won't let myself feel it. Maybe there is no terrible isolated event. Maybe it was something subtle, some daily nonverbal message that my mother had unknowingly conveyed to me. She didn't mean to; she was probably just repeating some pattern her mother had passed on to her."

I told Alexandra, "This is the heart of your story and your inability to conceive. By allowing yourself to feel what you actually experienced, you're coming to terms with what your parents did to you. In our work you have been seeing, naming, and feeling it." The critical voices of her internalized parents, which once shouted so loudly, were being stilled by Alexandra's growing sense of self-love. I said, "When you cry now, it's all of you feeling the sadness, not just one aspect of you. When you're joyful, the joy moves all through you. That's real freedom."

Alexandra found that one of the greatest benefits of her work in the Whole Person Fertility Program^{SM} was that her love relationship was even better than before. Although she had started the program saying that she and Cyril had an excellent relationship, she reported that they were closer now than they ever had been. Cyril had noted a change in her, especially the fact that she seemed to be calmer, happier, and less depressed. She found herself making time for them to be together, no matter how busy her professional life. They were developing a deeper level of intimacy.

The creation of new relationships with our parents is another positive outcome of the Whole Person Fertility Program^{SM}. We can feel greater love for our parents as we come to accept and understand that although they may have taught us negative love patterns, they did not create them. Renewing your relationship with your parents is actually an act of self-love because it allows you to achieve emotional independence. When we let go of fear and anger from the past, we cut the parental puppet strings. As Alexandra opened herself to the realities of her childhood, much of her rigidity abated, and she was able to develop a more comfortable connection with her parents.

As Alexandra continued working through her conscious and unconscious conflicts with her mother, she was moving closer to reconnecting with her inherent procreative power.

"I'm Pregnant!"

On the first of February, symbolically nine months after Alexandra and I had started our work together, she called and said, "I'm pregnant. I'm my new self—calmer, good, better. I'm leaving my old self behind. It's almost like I'm coming to my original self, before my parents distorted me." We both celebrated her announcement.

Alexandra gave birth to a healthy baby girl, Maria. I'll treasure the birth announcement and subsequent years of photos, as I do with all my clients who have conceived and birthed their babies. When I think of Alexandra, though, I will always remember the pen-and-ink drawing on my office wall, a gift from Alexandra, drawn by her when she was eight years old. It is symbolic of the work we did together. The image portrays a girl who is surrounded by sunlight and who is feeding birds. Birds symbolize the energy that brings about wholeness and balance with nature. The girl is the nurturing, powerful, loving Alexandra who always existed and who is now fused with the adult Alexandra, a young woman who will be consciously present to love, feed, and cuddle her newborn child.

Although Alexandra is one out of hundreds of my clients, each experience, including yours, is unique. You will find that by engaging in the exercises throughout the book, you will be helped to identify your personal history, as well as work toward resolving any emotional conflicts blocking conception. In this process, you will learn to express your true feelings, moving closer to connecting to your own self-loving nature and internal procreative wisdom.

FIVE

....

The Healing Journey

You have seen the Whole Person Fertility Pro-
gram^SM at work through Alexandra's story. Your
completion of the ephistogram and other preliminary exercises have laid the groundwork for the
Healing Journey on which we are about to embark
together. In the Healing Journey, you will actively engage in your own
healing process by identifying and releasing your repressed emotions
that can be inhibiting your ability to conceive. First, however, you need
to create a safe, nurturing environment for yourself through developing
your inner sanctuary and meeting your inner guide. You will then do
exercises that will help you discover your emotional reactions to experiences of which you may or may not be conscious. You also will become
more aware of the shadow side of yourself, which holds a great deal of
stored energy. By shadow I mean the parts of us that still are affected by
our painful childhood experiences. As you are confronting these
conception-blocking feelings through freeing, releasing exercises, you
are creating a new, emotionally open space that can respond to positive,
loving, fertile images. The steps in this unique program will help you
create a healthy emotional base from which you can move toward the
life you desire and deserve, and toward the life you will be creating.

I strongly recommend that you do not engage in this process

alone. The issues you are exploring are emotionally charged. Enlist the help of your mate, a trusted family member, or a nonjudgmental friend. You might suggest that they read this book as well—to help prepare them for the intensity of the process and to help them understand how and why it works. If you find that the support your mate or a friend provides is insufficient or uncomfortable for you, consider turning to a therapeutic professional, particularly one who has training and experience in emotional-release work. The highest aim of my work is to help you to mobilize your inner resources and strength by becoming your *own* healer. Of course, your past experiences will always be a part of you, but your consciousness of these experiences and how they affected you will make a crucial difference in how you work with and respond to them. That is where the healing occurs.

When I refer to a client's healing, I use words such as *beginning* and *becoming*. That's because the process of healing is ongoing. What I am suggesting is a new way to view life and to live it, not as a goal that needs to be reached within a finite period, but as a direction, a life intention. As you begin your own healing journey, you'll feel yourself moving three steps ahead, two back, and so forth as you continue to grow and heal.

Everything you have learned about yourself up to this point in *The Whole Person Fertility Program*^{SM} will be brought to bear in this chapter. The Healing Journey is an active process. It is an opportunity for you to discover your innermost strengths and resources for healing as you explore your family history and current life and their effect on your reproductive system.

Step 1: Creating Your Inner Sanctuary and Meeting Your Inner Guide

Every successful journey through uncharted territory needs a guide, and this first step is designed to make you your own inner guide. You'll use guided visual imagery—the mind thinking in pictures—to do this inner work. Imagery removes the constrictions of logical, linear thinking. To use imagery, we turn our attention inward to tap into the vast power of the mind-body to effect physical changes. As Dr. Dean Ornish has pointed out, "Your mind might think in words but your body responds to images as though they were really happening right now."[1]

When clients tell me they aren't good at visualizing, I generally suggest that they try the "fruit-tasting" exercise. This simple, popular exercise clearly demonstrates that one's imagination governs much of what one senses in one's body.

> Sit comfortably with your eyes closed. See yourself walking to the produce section of a supermarket. There are two bins in front of you: one filled with lemons and the other with oranges. Imagine yourself choosing a juicy yellow lemon. See yourself placing it on a cutting board that the market has provided. Now visualize yourself taking a sharp knife and cutting the lemon in half. Pick up the lemon and breathe in its lemony scent. Now visualize yourself sucking on the lemon. Feel your lips pucker at its sour taste. See yourself walking over to the bin of oranges. Pick one out and cut it in half, then quarters. Smell the sweet orange and then bite into a piece, allowing the juice to run down your chin. Feel yourself tasting the orange. Open your eyes.

This is an example of just how effective mental imagery can be. It can be sufficiently powerful to produce a state of relaxation essential to the conception process. You may want to record yourself reading the visualizations that follow or have someone you care for read the text to you—whichever approach makes you more comfortable. Hearing your own voice during the visualizations can reinforce the essential idea that you are becoming your own healer. Many guided visualizations, like the following ones, can produce the state of physical and mental relaxation that is essential to the conception and pregnancy process.

Most of us have become accustomed to looking outside ourselves for solace, support, love, and direction. While support from other people, such as a therapist, mate, family members, or friends is necessary, the most crucial support can come from within. Developing your sanctuary and inner guide as a part of the Healing Journey is essential in your healing process. Given the emotional depth of this process, you'll find that many feelings will be triggered and many long-forgotten memories unearthed that you alone can understand—with the help of your inner guide, who is available to you twenty-four hours a day. Your guide will always be supportive of you and will keep you centered throughout your journey.

An inner guide can be a teacher, a wise woman or wise man, an adviser, a religious figure, a friendly companion, or an animal. Connecting to your inner guide is a technique that has been used for centuries in many world cultures and religions. Deep down, you've probably always sensed this part of yourself. Perhaps you've heard its inner promptings and thought that if you paid more attention to this inner voice, you'd make better choices and be more effective in your life. Reflect back on some of the times you have ignored the advice of an inner voice and paid a price for not listening. Over the years, I have learned to stop, listen, and take appropriate action when I hear my inner guide speaking, even if it contradicts the best-intentioned advice of others. This exercise will help you do the same. Read through it once before you tape it.

TENSION-RELEASING/RELAXATION EXERCISE TO PREPARE FOR CREATING YOUR INNER SANCTUARY AND FINDING YOUR INNER GUIDE

1. Begin by selecting and playing music that you find quieting and conducive to reflection. Find a pillow, cushion, chair, or bed on which you can sit undisturbed for ten to twenty minutes. Sit in a comfortable position, positioning your body so that your head, neck, and spine are straight. Take a few slow, deep breaths in and out. Feel yourself quieting down. Close your eyes, if that is comfortable for you. Continue to take deep breaths, resting your

hands loosely on your lap—palms up—ready to receive and let
go of the tension in your body.

2. With each exhalation, release whatever tension is present in
   your body. There is no need to try to breathe deeply. Simply
   bring your attention to the natural rhythm of the inhalation and
   exhalation of your breath. Each time you notice your mind wandering from an awareness of the breath, gently and firmly direct
   your attention back to your belly, back to your breath. Now
   bring your awareness to the top of your head; take a deep breath
   and note if there is any tension present. With each exhalation,
   continue releasing that tension. Focus your attention on your
   eyes and jawline. Be mindful that your jawline is one of the
   major holding sites for a lot of tension. If you are experiencing
   any sensation of tightening or pain in your jaw, ask yourself
   whether you are feeling angry. If so, note what the anger may be
   about while gently rubbing your jaw and relaxing your facial
   muscles.

3. As you continue breathing, visualize your right and left shoulders. Note if there is tension present in your shoulders or neck.
   Now move your awareness from your right shoulder down your
   arm to your right hand. Release any tension through your fingertips by seeing yourself opening five tiny golden faucets, one on
   each fingertip, letting the tension flow out, and then closing the
   faucets.

4. Take another deep breath and shift your awareness to the left side
   of your body. Beginning with your left shoulder and moving
   down your arm and hand, release any tension by opening the
   tiny golden faucet on each fingertip and allowing the tension to
   drain off, then closing the faucets. Now bring your awareness to
   your chest and note if there is any tension or tightness, and then
   down your abdomen, your back, and your buttocks....Note if

your breathing is shallow or full. Now direct your attention to your genital area. Take several deep breaths and release any tension in that area.

5. Move your awareness down the right side of your body from the hip, down the legs and to the toes. Again, release any tension through the tiny golden faucet on each of your five toes. Shift to the left side of your body, slowly moving down and releasing all the tension on your left side out of the tiny faucet on each toe of your left foot, continuing to be mindful of your breathing.

Creating Your Inner Sanctuary

Now, in your imagination think of a place in which you feel safe, joyful, peaceful, and relaxed. Your sanctuary could be a special room in your home, a favorite beach by the ocean, an overlook or glen in the mountains, or any place that evokes warm, comforting memories and feelings for you. This is your sanctuary, your private space. Take a few deep breaths and visualize this place in as much detail as you can, invoking all of your senses. What do you see? What do you hear and smell? Are there flowers? What colors do you see? Does your sanctuary have any specific shape? Are there trees? Is there water? Are there birds? Animals? Take time to pay attention to all of the details of your sanctuary, because they will be important for you as this experience progresses. As you recall your safe space, if a negative memory pops up, don't push it away. Take a deep breath and gently bring your awareness back to the place where you feel safe and cared for. Know that at any moment when you feel tense or face a situation that is difficult for you to handle, you can visualize yourself back in your sanctuary, releasing any tension or discomfort you are holding in your body. My sanctuary is a beautiful scallop-shaped beach in Costa Rica, filled with a vast array of magnificently colored shells. As a seashell collector, this is my paradise—now in my imagination.

Meeting Your Inner Guide

Remaining in a meditative, reflective, relaxed state, sit in your inner sanctuary and keep your eyes closed. Focus on your breathing. Now you can begin to connect with your inner guide. Realize that this inner guide has always been there for you. Allow yourself to feel whatever comes up as you open to meeting this guide who will continue to always be with you.

Now picture yourself walking around your sanctuary. You may see a figure, someone or something that's coming into view. It may be a woman, man, animal, or even an inanimate object, a touchstone, or someone you have known and whom you trust completely. Does this figure feel familiar to you? If this figure is a man or a woman, how is he or she dressed? If the figure you meet does not feel friendly or is too judgmental, ask yourself who might that person be. You can keep walking around in your sanctuary until you find the wise person or guide who you want and who is offering you love, compassion, and understanding. In your mind's eye, anything is possible. This is your sanctuary, and although no one can enter without your permission, negative internal images may be there from the past. This time, though, you have a choice. If you visualize this negative figure, see it walking off into the distance, or, with a touch of your finger, you can make it disappear in a cloud of smoke.

Keep on with your search until you meet the wise, loving figure you want for yourself. When you do, take a deep breath, be mindful of any tension in your body, and release that tension. Lead your guide to a place in your sanctuary where you can talk together. Feel how wonderful it is to be in the presence of someone who loves you unconditionally, knows you completely, and who can give you the answers to your most pressing questions.

One possible question you may ask is: "What information do you have for me that I am not paying attention to?" Listen to the response. If you are going through a difficult time trying to become pregnant, or if a pregnancy did not hold or a medical procedure did not work, your inner guide is ideal for you to talk to. You may ask any question and then wait for a response. If the guide does not answer immediately, while you are still in the sanctuary, look for a response from an unanticipated external source as the days unfold. Sometimes a response can come in the form of a letter, phone call, magazine article, a song, or it might grow out of your continued work in this chapter or other chapters in this book. Have patience—at first allow yourself just to connect with your guide—trust and stay open, receptive to receiving information. It may take time. Practice patience.

If you have not found your inner guide at this point, ask yourself what your guide looks like. Don't get discouraged; just try this visualization again, remaining as open as possible to answers. Many of us are unaware that the real vitality is in the questions, which keep you open to new possibilities. Conscious and unconscious messages race between our brain and nervous system at the speed of 185 miles per hour. Someone once estimated that at least one thousand messages each day come from our inner guide but we often don't hear the voice within. Imagine how your life will improve now that you are becoming open and receptive, ready to listen to your inner guide.

Know that whenever you need to, you will be able to enter your inner sanctuary and hear the voice of your inner guide: coaxing, whispering, singing words of love and wisdom, words of illumination and wonder—always there, continuing to offer direction throughout your healing journey. When you are ready, open your eyes and take a deep breath, bringing your awareness back into the room.

After you emerge from this experience, draw your sanctuary on paper, using crayons, colored markers or pencils, paints, or watercolors. Fill in as many of the details as possible, including your guide, if you have found one, the place, flowers, trees—drawing all these details can make your sanctuary come alive and make it more real for you. Note the colors you have used. Do they have meaning for you? Place your drawing in a readily accessible area, maybe next to your bed, so you see it when you go to sleep and when you first wake in the morning, as a reminder of what is available for you. You will find that your inner guide can be extremely helpful as you cope with situations regarding your difficulties in conceiving.

Step 2: Exploring Your Attitudes Toward Pregnancy and Childbirth

Answering the following questions will stimulate thoughts, feelings, and concerns about pregnancy and childbirth, and where these attitudes might have originated. On a clean page in your journal, write down your responses.

1. What did you hear about pregnancy and childbirth as you were growing up?
2. What did your mother tell you about her experiences conceiving, carrying, and delivering you and your siblings?
3. Specifically, what did you hear about your birth?
4. Was your mother working at the time of her conception and what was her age? Did your mother continue or stop working after your birth? Was it work that she enjoyed? Did her work represent the fulfillment of her life's dream—or not? What did she tell you about it? What feelings does this evoke in you? Did she ever discuss her feelings with you?
5. Are you being pressured to have a child? By whom? How do you feel about this?
6. Do you have any concerns about conception? What did you hear about pregnancy, childbirth, and parenting, and from whom?

When you return to your sanctuary again, talk with your inner guide about the key areas that came up for you in answering these questions. What do you feel you need to address on your journey to conception?

Step 3: Photoanalysis: Looking into the Windows of Your Past to Understand Your Present

As we discussed earlier, family photographs can be powerful tools in documenting our past, reminding us of where we have been and how we have developed emotionally as well as physically. This exercise is based on the work of Dr. Robert U. Akert, whose book *Photoanalysis* (New York: Peter H. Wyden, Inc., 1973) introduced his theory that photographs are psychological treasures. Comparing them to dreams, body language, and handwriting, he found that photographs "contain clues invisible to the untrained eye: the true meaning of smiles, hands, groupings, poses, distances between people, why your little brother never looked at the camera; who was your grandmother's favorite grandchild."

Once you begin looking at your photographs from the point of view of understanding your family's dynamics, you'll never view a snapshot in quite the same way again. As an essential element in my initial consultation, I ask clients to bring in photos of themselves with family members.

Whether you have one hundred photos or just a few, they can be extremely helpful. Select a group of photographs of yourself at various ages and stages of life—with family members, your mate, animals, and so on. Body-language characteristics are evident from a very young age and reveal our ease or discomfort with life as we grew up.

If any of the photos you have chosen to analyze evoke strong feelings for you, allow yourself to experience them. Here are a few guidelines to help you analyze:

1. Look at who is standing or sitting next to whom. Are these seating arrangements repeated in other photos? Is someone usually outside the group? Is someone usually in the middle?

2. Are there spaces between you and other family members? Are there spaces between one family member and another? Who seems relaxed, perhaps because they are lounging in a

comfortable position? Does anyone have his or her arms around another person? Is anyone touching? Who seems tense? Are some people sitting formally, with their hands clasped in their laps or with their arms held rigidly by their sides? (If you are looking at old photographs—say, of your grandparents' generation—keep in mind that formality was the custom for taking photographs, so the above details might not be true indicators.)

3. What do your facial expressions convey to you? Sadness? Happiness? Joy? Anger? Can you recall feeling special? Excluded? What are the similarities in the way you felt then that are still true now? What are the differences?

4. What facial expressions do your parents have? What can you tell about your parents' relationship to each other from the photos? Do you notice any similarities or differences between what you can read in their relationship and your own relationship with your mate today? What are they?

5. What are the facial expressions of your siblings? Is there a sibling who often seems to be receiving more parental attention or who is often excluded from the family? Who looks happy? Sad? Angry? What can you now read in looking at your siblings that still holds true for them today? How do you feel about this?

6. How are babies regarded in the photos? Are they cradled lovingly or are they held away from the mother's or father's body?

As one example of how important these photos are and how they can be used in my process, one of my clients brought in a snapshot of her mother leaving the hospital after her birth. Her mother's arms were outstretched, holding my client at arm's length, seemingly without any of the innate common sense that leads us to cradle and support a baby's head. The client said, "My mother looks as if she's trying to drop me. I know my sense of not being wanted has a basis in reality. It wasn't my imagination."

7. Choose the one childhood photograph of yourself that seems to leap out at you. Speak to yourself in this picture as if you could go back in time and whisper words of love and reassurance. Tell

yourself whatever it was that you needed to hear then and still need to hear in order to heal. When you have finished speaking, summarize the words into one sentence. Write them down on a slip of paper and place this over your mirror or in your journal—somewhere you will see it every day.

Sue, a client, found one of her baby pictures that had been taken when she was eight months old—shortly after her father had deserted her mother. The photo painfully reminded her that her mother then left her in another state for two years to be raised by an eighteen-year-old aunt. She said to her eight-month-old self, "I can hear Mommy telling you to smile. But you seemed to want to cry. That's why you have that half smile on your face. You had no reason to be happy, and you knew it." Sue's credo became: Express what you truly feel.

Step 4: Touring the Crowded Childhood Rooms of Your Mind

This visualization exercise helps you to go back in time to reexperience feelings as well as hidden memories of childhood that may be affecting your efforts to conceive today. You need to give yourself at least a half hour to participate in the following exercise effectively. You may want to record your voice reading this exercise aloud.

1. Sit in a quiet, private place, eyes closed. Begin to focus on your breathing and take several deep, cleansing breaths. Inhale deeply and as fully as you can comfortably, pause, and then exhale slowly. Know that with each inhalation you are taking into your body oxygen that cleanses and heals. Take another deep breath and send it down into your belly. Breathe out as fully as possible. Know that with every exhalation you are cleansing your body of toxins.

2. See yourself going down five steps—taking deep breaths one step at a time; as you get to the bottom, you see there is a long silvery

tunnel. See yourself entering the tunnel at the age and size that
you are. Now notice that as you proceed through the tunnel you
become younger and younger as you move along, until you are
at the earliest age and size you remember yourself.

3. As you come out of the tunnel, see yourself standing in front of
the door to the house or apartment in which you grew up. Take
note of what you are feeling. If you are aware of any tension in
your body, take a deep breath and release it. Be mindful of all
the emotional and physical feelings that are bound to crop up
as you go back into your childhood experiences. What age are
you? What are you wearing? What does your face look like?
What is your earliest memory that you can recall in that house?
Does it feel painful? Bad? Joyous? Now see yourself opening
the door. What is the first image that greets you? Note your
reaction to whatever that image might be. As you're walking
into the house or apartment, ask yourself where you slept.
Where was your bedroom in relation to your mother and
father's? Did they sleep in the same bedroom, or did they have
separate rooms? Take a deep breath and be aware of any tension as you move forward. How did your parents relate?
Warmly? With hostility? Sexually? Nonsexually? Was your
father or mother away a good deal of the time? Did you have to
share your bedroom with a sibling? Which one? What was that
experience like? Did any of your parents' siblings (your aunts
and uncles) live with you? Which ones? What was your relationship to the relatives? Do you know why they lived with you,
if they did?

4. See yourself wandering around the kitchen, living room, dining
room—if there was one—and note your reactions to whatever
you can recall in each room. Can you see your mother in the
house? Your father? Where are they? What are they doing? Does
your vision of your parents bring up any feelings for you? What

do you see them doing? Can you make eye contact with your mother? With your father? What do you see? Stay as closely in touch with what comes up for you as you travel through the rooms of your childhood house. And take deep breaths. Did you have any pets? Was there a play area? Was play encouraged in your house? Or did you have to be very quiet? How many bathrooms were there? Was that a problem? How much time did your mother spend with you? Your father? What do you see yourself doing with your siblings? How do you feel when you imagine your mother? Your father? Your siblings? Do you get any visceral responses? Keep walking through the rooms, looking again at your bedroom and noting all the feelings that come up for you. Was it a room you liked to be in? Or did you not like to be there? Why?

5. See if you can tune in to any conversations you hear going on in the childhood rooms of your mind. Did your parents argue? What did that feel like for you? Did your maternal or paternal grandparents live with you? What did that feel like? How did your mother get along with her mother? Her father? How did your father get along with his parents? Did you play any games with your siblings? Was there a garden available to play in? Did the house have trees, plants, or flowers? In your mind's eye, do they appear cared for? What were the rules of the house? Did you all have to show up for dinner at the same time? Were you allowed to cry? To be angry? Do you feel that your mother enjoyed you and your siblings? Did your father? How? Who was the favorite sibling? Who was the least-favored sibling? As a child, were you to be seen and not heard?

6. Keep walking through the rooms and seeing whatever additional memories might be triggered as you revisit your childhood home. Was there any physical abuse? If there was, what do you recall about the experience either for you or your siblings? Look and see how your siblings related to one another. Were you the

insider or the outsider? Try to recall every experience possible, both joyful and painful. Was there a rigid structure with high expectations, and how do you feel about that? How did you feel then and how do you feel now when recalling these experiences? See if the questions above stimulated other questions that you might wish to explore.

7. As you begin to reenter the tunnel, see yourself slowly moving forward along this long silvery tunnel, getting older and older as you move toward the front, toward the opening of the tunnel, toward the present. Give yourself as much time as you need. Slowly bring yourself away from these childhood experiences. How do you feel as you leave? What's being triggered emotionally and physically? Be mindful of your breathing and continue walking. See the tunnel getting larger and larger to accommodate the age and size you are right now. As you are moving out of the tunnel, see the staircase of five steps. Begin your climb back up. Take a deep breath and begin counting, one, two, three, four—and as you are about to approach the fifth step, slowly bring your consciousness back into the present room.

8. Take some time to write in your journal as many of your remembrances as you can. As you look back at this experience, what was the most joyful part? What was the most painful? Note if you have any other questions. What you are looking for are patterns of behavior that existed in your home life as a child that you now may see embodied in your thoughts, beliefs, attitudes, and behaviors affecting your sexual and reproductive life. Give yourself a hug for the courage to have traveled back in time and to have allowed yourself to reexperience feelings that were painful. If you would like, go into your sanctuary, your inner healing space, and sit there for a while, perhaps talking with your inner guide about your experiences. Consider sharing these experiences with your mate.

Step 5: Pillow Talk

Pillow talk is one of the most important emotional-release techniques in the Whole Person Fertility Program.^{SM} I recommend its use for releasing repressed emotions in a variety of situations. I used this process with Alexandra, whose story appeared in chapter 4, and still do with many of my clients. Alexandra, like most of my clients, utilized pillow talk to confront her parents imaginarily about unresolved emotional issues she had with them. This exercise is particularly useful if you cannot confront a person in your life with whom you have a conflict. It is also useful to practice talking out your issues if you intend to confront someone, so that you have a clear sense of what you may want to tell them face-to-face. You can use this exercise as needed to release a whole range of thoughts, feelings, and emotions.

1. Designate pillows as stand-ins for significant people in your life with whom you have a conflict (e.g., family, friends, mate, boss, or coworkers).

2. Locate a focal point of your pain so you can begin releasing your powerful, potentially damaging emotions. Begin speaking to the pillow or pillows as you wish you could in person. Give yourself free range—don't censor yourself. This exercise is for you—to release your emotions, whatever they are, however embarrassing, shocking, rageful, or disturbing they may be. Release any guilt you have—what you are doing cannot hurt anyone's feelings because you are doing this in the privacy of your space to help you heal.

3. Remember to "take your pain home." No matter who legitimately may be the target of your strong emotions, understand how those feelings connect to childhood experiences. That's the direction

your symptoms and your emotions are pointing to. Your body and your mind want relief, and in taking charge of your healing, you begin to give your mind-body exactly what it is asking for.

4. Speak as long as you want to, until you feel as if you have drained your emotional well. When you are done, you may feel that you want to reconcile with a specific person through the pillow. You can hug the pillow, comforting and consoling yourself.

Though at first you may feel uncomfortable doing this exercise because you feel as if you are playacting, it will become more real for you as you continue to engage in the process. Keep in mind that this is a portable exercise. It can be used whenever you are alone and can shut a door for some privacy. If you feel inexplicable sadness, anger, or any physical symptom manifesting, you can release the tension in your body—tension that may have been exacerbated by past hurts—through pillow talk.

Judith, a client who now describes herself as a "pillow talk aficionado," was at home the night before a celebration in honor of her being made a partner in a prestigious law firm, when she suddenly developed an excruciating stomachache. The first thing she did was ask herself, "What is going on? Why am I 'aching my stomach' at the very moment when I've become that success I'd always wanted to be?" She realized that she was feeling angry, but didn't know why. As she was questioning what her stomach pains could be about, she thought of Sally, one of the senior women in the firm, who she felt was extremely aggravating. She designated a pillow to be Sally, who would be at the celebration. Sally rarely acknowledged Judith and was always critical of her.

Judith started talking to her Sally pillow, saying, "Why are you robbing me of this moment? You're so hard on me, I can't even accept my achievement without aching my stomach." Through her work with me, Judith knew to link her current anger to her childhood experiences. She shouted at the pillow, "Who are you?" After a moment, she asked, "You're Dad, aren't you? Dad was who never showed up for my school awards, no matter how well I did. But you were always there for my brothers, even for the damn Boy Scout meetings." She began to cry, feeling the aloneness of being a little girl on the stage and winning the state spelling bee. "I felt so alone in my achievements," she said. Judith was amazed that after only five minutes of pillow talk, her stomach pains were gone. The next day she fully enjoyed the award ceremony.

Don't be afraid to improvise. One client told me how she used emotional-release work while focusing on a steering wheel. Another—the owner of a shoe store—insisted that she be the one, not her employees, to tear up the packaging boxes for recycling. "It's the time of the day I really look forward to," she said. If there are other people within hearing range—in a ladies' room, for instance—try going into a stall and silently but furiously tearing paper towels into shreds. When you've finished, flush those feelings away. Some of my clients who enjoy swimming have found that they can release strong emotions by splashing the water. Another client goes to her health club and uses a punching bag to let loose. A teenager I know uses the plastic grocery bags stored beneath the kitchen sink to kick these surrogate parents across his bedroom.

What's key in all of these efforts is your skillful use of your energy. To get angry with the right person, to the right degree, at the right time, for the right purpose, and in the right way requires knowledge and self-awareness. As you become physically engaged in the exercise, it's also important whenever possible that you continue to communicate your feelings verbally. As you continue to broaden your pillow-talk techniques, give a voice to this person with whom you are upset—allow him or her to answer back through you. You can clarify what you really are upset about as you listen to what this person has to say about you.

Step 6: Reconnecting with Mother

Just as children turn to their mothers for recognition, wanting to be just like them when they grow up, so do grown women yearn for their mother's basic approval and understanding (which most feel they did not receive). As one client wrote to her mother, "I feel as though I have been beating on the locked door of your heart, getting you to open up to hear me."

The women of the baby boom generation are caught in an intense conflict of wanting the "little girl" recognition while at the same time actively rejecting their mother's life. Bringing this conflict to consciousness frees blocked energy.

The major breakthrough occurs when you change your consciousness and instead of saying, "I don't want to be anything like you," repeatedly ask, "How am I like you?" This lays the foundation for clearly understanding what you need to separate from and to reconnect to in the past in order to create a new life for yourself today.

The willingness to understand your childhood pain and bring these experiences to consciousness helps you relate to your mother's pain and heal your relationship with yourself and your mother. Ultimately, we need to come to terms, hopefully lovingly, with our mothers, reaching a point at which we neither feel alienated from ourselves nor hate vital aspects of our feminine bodies and our reproductive system.

Confronting these hurtful experiences allows the light of healing to enter—forgiving our parents does not mean forgiving any hurts they may have caused us. I realize at times it is hard to separate the two. The Amish say, "You forgive the abuser but not the abuse." This exercise is powerful to experience whether your mother is alive or not.

1. Select a piece of music you love that touches your heart and soul. Soften the lighting with candles if appropriate. Remove any distractions—for example, turn down the ringer on the phone.

2. Sit comfortably and close your eyes. Go to your inner sanctuary (see "Step 1" on page 126) and invite your mother to join you.

3. Picture yourself sitting facing your mother and making eye contact. Look deeply into each other's eyes. What are you seeing? Is she maintaining eye contact with you? Do her eyes convey any feelings? Where are her arms and hands? Where are yours? Notice her body language. How is she sitting? Is she inviting you in, or do you feel she is locking you out?

4. Allow yourself to experience fully whatever emotions are present, even if they are uncomfortable or upsetting.

5. Tell her all of the negative things she has told you about pregnancy and childbirth that are still upsetting you today.

6. Explain to your mother what you understand and feel about not becoming pregnant.

7. At some point, listen carefully to what you imagine or want her response to be. Realize how in describing your efforts not to be like her you also may have rejected her reproductive ability.

8. Imagine taking her hands in yours and expressing what you feel needs healing between you in order to reclaim your right to have your baby. Have your mother respond as you would like her to. Leave your inner sanctuary together. When you reach the exit, take with you the reproductive and fertile aspects of your mother that you need in order to conceive.

Following this experience, write a letter to your mom—whether you choose to mail it or not—about what you are feeling. If you can have this dialogue with her personally, that would be wonderful, but remember, this is not about changing her. This is about your right to express your feelings, reclaiming and freeing your personal and reproductive power.

Step 7: Reparenting Your Inner Child

We can reparent our inner child by recognizing its needs and responding with acceptance, love, and affection to her or him. The child within refers to that part of each of us that is alive, energetic, creative, and fulfilled; it is our real self—who we truly are. It's the delightful, childlike part of us.

Seeking to conceive often brings us back to our early, painful childhood experiences filled with unresolved conflicts, unmet needs, deep longings, and rage. Many of my clients are either resistant to or angry with their "little self," blaming her or him for their feeling badly. Most of us are unaware that our internalized parents' negative, judgmental feelings are acting against our inner child's needs and well-being.

We learn to reparent by recognizing and legitimizing our inner child's needs, which allows us to reconnect with the full range of our feelings: the light and the dark; the joy and the wonderment; the anger, pain, and sorrow. Healing that inner part of us that needs to be affirmed, appreciated, heard, and understood moves us into the wonderment of the childlike state of being, which is crucial to the process of creative conscious conception.

I have found the following exercise, as part of my experience in the Hoffman Training Program, to be extremely helpful. In reconnecting with your full range of feelings, you will become aware of your inner child, thus allowing it to mature. Do this exercise every night for several weeks.

1. Find a comfortable place to sit in your sanctuary. Place two pillows on the floor, one representing you and one representing the "little self" part of you. Close your eyes and take several deep breaths as you slowly become more centered. Quiet your breathing as you slowly release any tension you may be holding. Open your eyes and begin a dialogue with your inner child, asking questions such as:

    a. What was your day like?

    b. How are you feeling? Happy? Sad? Anxious? Lonely?

    c. How can I help you?

    d. What would you like to do today?

    e. How about having some fun?

2. Listen—really listen—by switching places back and forth and letting your inner child speak to you without you responding.

3. Take several deep breaths and allow yourself to relax and stay connected with your inner child. Is she or he feeling anxious and uneasy, or relaxed? Begin to see that the anxious and uneasy inner child is not all of you but only one part of you. Realize that this part of you—the wounded little girl or boy—is no longer alone. Let yourself breathe through the anxiety, not denying it but acknowledging the anxiety. Take another deep breath and rub your belly, addressing your inner child: "I feel your anxiety and your uneasiness, but I am here now; I am here to help you get through whatever it is you are feeling."

As one client said to me, "My mother was too absorbed in her own painful life to be truly present for me. I understand that now. But I can take charge and be that parent for myself—present for my inner child's delightful childlike exuberance and joy—as well as the times she is feeling anxious, fearful, and tense. I will rub her belly, tell her how much I love her, reassuring her that I'm present and that I understand what she is feeling. It is amazing how quieting this experience is."

Step 8: Grief Ceremony: Mourning Miscarriage, Abortion, and Stillbirth

To facilitate the grieving process, I created this heartfelt ceremony to allow you consciously to mourn your losses and emotionally release your unborn child. Although there is one basic ceremony, I am quite aware that each circumstance carries with it different emotions. For instance, a woman who has had a miscarriage obviously has a different set of feelings and energy from a woman who may have lost a sibling or who is grieving an abortion. If your child was unborn, it is vital that you acknowledge the loss as a real one. Whether you experienced your loss recently or decades earlier, this ceremony will allow you to validate your sorrow.

Another client once said that she worried she would "cry too much" if she participated in a ritualized ceremony. Whether tears are an expression of sorrow, anger, or joy, they typically make people feel uncomfortable. Crying out one's pain is what I call "God's inner bath." Unfortunately, growing up, many of us were not encouraged to feel and express our emotions. Crying actually produces relaxation chemicals in your body that can alter your biochemistry in a positive way and help your body to release toxins. Dr. Stephen Bloomfield believes tears allow our bodies to lower tension levels. By holding back our tears, we contain our pain, which negatively affects the body. Tears are crucial to our physical and emotional health—a benefit that so many of my clients have experienced during their grief ceremonies.

There are many ways to express your grief. One of my clients held her ceremony on a windy hillside and used a paper kite to represent her unborn child. At the end of the ceremony, she released the kite and watched as it was carried out over the Pacific Ocean. Using this method is best done in a wide open area away from any trees so your balloon or kite won't get stuck before it has a chance to fly skyward. Feel free to use the instructions below as guidelines for creating your personal grief ceremony.

1. To prepare for a formalized grief ceremony, purchase a lifelike infant doll (a cushion or pillow can substitute for the doll) and a receiving blanket. You will need white candles and flowers, meditative music, and soft cushions for sitting. You may want to invite your mate or a close, supportive friend or relative to participate in this service with you.

2. Before you begin the ceremony, write a letter to your unborn child that you will then read aloud during the ceremony. Whether or not you choose to conduct the full grief ceremony, writing a letter to your unborn child will allow you to tap into your deeper feelings. Your mate may also wish to write one. If you chose a name for your unborn child, address the letter with that name. If not, you may want to address him or her as your "dearly missed child." (I am using "him" to designate both

sexes.) Explain to your child why his life was important to you, how you feel about his loss, and why you are writing this letter. Also tell him why you feel it is necessary to release him, so that his soul can travel on, perhaps to a home ready to receive him. You may want to add that should his spirit return to you when you are ready to receive him, you will be grateful. Conclude your letter with words that will help you feel a sense of closure, such as "Good-bye [adding the child's name]. I will never forget you." After you have completed your letter, you can begin your grief ceremony when you are ready to do so. Be kind, nurturing, and patient with yourself and your feelings.

3. Place the vase of white flowers beside the white candles in candle holders. As you light the candles, lower the lights in the room. With gentle and reflective music playing in the background, place your infant doll, wrapped in a receiving blanket, on a cushion, with the candles illuminating your "baby." Remain aware of your feelings as you go through the preparation for the ceremony and continue to breathe deeply, releasing any tension you might be holding in your body.

4. Sit comfortably and exhale as deeply as you can. You as well as those who are present can participate in the following visualization:

Envision yourself in a beautiful meadow. The birds are singing and the sun is warm, deeply penetrating all of life in and around you. Allow yourself to go into this meditative state. You might want to read a prayer of your choice, or you could read this prayer, called "the Gayatri,"[2] which embodies the spirit of Wholeness. Address the sun in this fashion: "You, who are the source of all power, Whose rays illuminate the whole world, Illuminate also my heart so that it too can do Your Work." While reciting the Gayatri, visualize the sun's rays streaming forth into the world, entering into your heart, and then streaming out from your heart's center back into the world. This is a powerful and life-enhancing prayer.

5. Read aloud the letter that you have written to your unborn child. If you have a mate or friend present, allow yourself to be comforted and physically supported. If not, wrap your arms around yourself, giving yourself a hug.

6. At the culmination of your reading, pick up the blanketed "baby" and cradle it in your arms. As your ceremony ends, realize that this is the first step in opening yourself to your pain, grief, and healing.

Lia's story shows how one woman's grief ceremony over her past abortions helped her to heal very deep and painful wounds.

Lia, a thirty-nine-year-old TV news executive, had learned not to cry, because in her family it was seen as being "wimpy." She began her grief ceremony dry-eyed. She started by addressing the deep sense of shame that she had been struggling with over her two previous abortions. As Lia became more comfortable with the process, she began to verbalize the self-blame she had been carrying. I gently encouraged her to take several deep breaths as she unearthed the pain that she had buried so deep within her psyche and the cells of her body.

Lia voiced the core dilemma in which many working women have found themselves. Concerning her choices, Lia said, "I had decided that I wouldn't be like my sisters, who were housewives and who seemed to live for their husbands and children. I was the news director, responsible for determining what and how information would be disseminated throughout one of the most important cities of the world. That used to sound so important, but it pales in comparison to what my sisters have known: the love of babies; holding your daughter's hand as she takes her first step. I can't forgive myself for my abortions. I distanced myself from my sisters' lives by putting them down. Now I'm the failure. I'm the one who can't admit to them that I've had two abortions. I'd rather they see me as infertile. I don't want them to know I want children, because I've made such a big deal about not wanting them. Now I want those two souls back."

Forgetting her proscription against tears, Lia wept despondently. After a few minutes, she felt strong enough to address her two "babies," who were lying wrapped in receiving blankets. She said through her tears, "God has forgiven me, and I hope you will, too. I made the wrong decision and now I want your two souls to come back to me. I feel so bad that I had to make you wait so long. But I wasn't ready to be a mother to you yet. I would have raised you the same way I was raised, and that my mother was raised, and her mother before her. I want you to give me another chance. I've been working hard on releasing the pain that was passed down to me. And Henrik would be a good daddy to you....But I want you to know that even if you don't come back to us, I hope you will go to another mom and dad, parents who want you and can be good to you....I know I must release you. I love you and I have to let you go to open space in me for a new pregnancy."

Lia lifted the dolls and hugged them to her breasts. "Good-bye, my loves. I know that God is with you." As she kissed each "child," she said, "I really need you. I really love you. Please come back. God be with you." We wept together.

Now that you have begun the difficult work of releasing so many powerful emotions, such as your unexpressed grief from engaging in the preceding emotional-release ceremony, begin to visualize your inherent, fertile being. The following exercises will assist you in seeing yourself as a vibrant woman whose generative powers spring from her very essence.

Step 9: Nature's Ode to Conception

This visualization is specifically designed to celebrate your fertility and to help prepare your endometrium, the mucous membrane lining the uterus, to receive a fertilized egg and hold the pregnancy to term.

You can either have your mate or a friend read the following to you or you can read it aloud into a tape recorder, accompanied by reflective music that you find soothing and comforting.

Begin by making yourself comfortable, shifting your weight so you can feel fully supported, whether you are sitting or lying down.

Let your eyes gently close. Note if your head, neck, and spine are in alignment. Take a cleansing breath; inhale as fully as you can, pause, and then breathe out. Take another deep breath and as you exhale imagine you are sending it down into your belly. Take another deep breath and as you exhale send the warm energy of your breath to any part of your body that feels sore, tense, or tight. As you continue breathing deeply, release any tension with each exhalation. Feel your body slowly ease and relax, loosening and letting go of all tense areas. Allow yourself to feel safe and comfortable, relaxed and easy.

Now picture yourself in a beautiful forest. The forest is the abundant fertility of the primordial Earth Mother. It is rich with dark green foliage. Overhead there is a brilliant, warm sun. Take a deep breath. The blue sky is crystal clear. As you walk through this lush, highly vegetated green forest, there is an underlying green moss carpet spread on the rich soil. This forest is so fertile with life, so abundant with life. Listen to the excitement of the birds singing, calling to one another in the sweetest symphony in the world. It is nature's symphony, an ode to life, an ode to creation, an ode to fertility. In your mind's eye, see an absolutely exquisite sun. Visualize the sun's rays streaming forth through the foliage of the trees, entering your heart and warming every space within your being. See the rays then streaming out of your heart's center and back into the world. Listen to the birds singing a song of fertility, of life, renewal of life; just listen for a few moments. Breathe deeply.

You can hear a brook somewhere in the distance, flowing over the rocks and twigs, adding its sounds to the most exquisite symphony of sound and movement. Now…see beautiful white, pink, and orchid flowers. Look at their colors as you breathe in their fragrances, sending the essence down into your womb, opening, receiving, and giving forth. The sun is continuing to send its healing rays throughout every cell, tissue, and muscle of your body, bringing its rays right into your womb.

As you feel the warmth of the sun's rays penetrating deeply into your uterus, see the rays streaming forth from your womb out into the world, healing the world. There is a beautiful circular energy pulsating throughout—into your body, then out, into your body and out. Every part of your body feels so relaxed. As with all of nature, your body is ready to receive and give forth, receive and give forth.

In the midst of this wonderful process of receiving and letting go, realize that anytime there are feelings of sadness, anger, tension, worry, anxiety, they, too, are part of nature. Nature is not only sun; it is also wind, rain, and storms. Nature is hurricanes, tornadoes, floods, and blizzards. All of this is nature. Add some protection from the storms of life for the new life you want to grow within you. See yourself placing your future baby in a beautiful pink bubble. This isn't just any pink bubble: it's an exquisite crystalline bubble that is full of life-enhancing oxygen to protect the baby for the moments when you experience emotional reactions to difficult situations. You can say to the baby, "I'm here to protect you. I can't promise that I will be the world's best mom. I will make mistakes. I will not have cleansed everything negative from my psyche, but I welcome your arrival and I am committed to doing my very best." When you feel you are ready, slowly open your eyes.

After this visualization, write down in your journal your own message to your future baby with a prayer that the spirit and the body unite to form the creation of the baby you have long waited for.

Step 10: Circle of Light Ceremony

In your journal, write down all of the things that you feel you deserve to have and what you will attain. To envision yourself experiencing this future life in which you have all that you want and need, create a circle of light ceremony. Place a circle of lit candles around you. Sit comfortably in the middle. Breathe deeply and relax. The warmth and glow of the candles represents a circle of protection, autonomy, and freedom from guilt about getting what you need and want. Read aloud all that you plan to attain. Try to picture these things clearly in your mind. Experience whatever emotions you have that accompany these visions. When you have completed this ritual, extinguish the candles. At least once a day for the next week—while you are in the shower, walking during the day, or before going to bed—recall the glow of the candles and this vision of the life you deserve.

In your mind's eye, see yourself radiating perfect health—see every cell in your body illuminated and your reproductive system healthy and vibrant. Visualize your life exactly as you wish it to be.

In your mind's eye, see and feel yourself living your highest dreams. If there is anything you want, see it already as your reality.

No Endings, Only New Beginnings

The end of this chapter is not the end of your healing journey. These exercises can be done anytime you feel you need them in support of your journey. I especially encourage you to practice "Step 9: Nature's Ode to Conception" often—when trying to conceive and after, while your new baby is either anticipated or in your womb. Continue working through the rest of the book, even if you do not have the specific reproductive difficulties addressed in Part Three. Each chapter contains valuable information that will guide you on your journey.

PART THREE

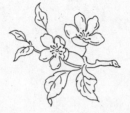

*Emotional Keys
to Healing Specific
Reproductive Issues*

SIX

·····················

Communicating with Your Mind-Body

Physical symptoms are wake-up calls that indicate something in your life needs your attention. Underlying virtually every physical condition and symptom are bottled-up thoughts, feelings, and emotional reactions. When you are willing to listen to the messages your symptoms convey to you, there is an opportunity to heal your life as well as your mind-body.

Think of your body as your ally who is sending you symptoms as messages about your life—what is not working as you would like it to work and what you need to change. To learn to listen to your body, you need to be aware of the connection between your thoughts and feelings (e.g., anger, anxiety, fear, sadness) and physiological responses (e.g., muscle tension, cold hands, or an accelerated heartbeat). Think, for instance, of how you feel in anticipation of seeing someone you love. Notice how your body reacts. Now think of how your body feels when you imagine yourself back in an argument you had with someone a long time ago. Finally, think of a special place where you feel at peace and relaxed. This is the kind of mind-body awareness you need to bring to the symptoms your body is expressing.

You will find that it is easier to maintain a mind-body awareness when you explore the meaning of your symptoms by learning how to question yourself in a different way from how you usually do. For example, when you have a stomachache, you need to ask yourself, Why am I aching my stomach? or What is aching my stomach? If you have indigestion, you might ask, What in my life is indigestible for me? Or if you have severe cramps before menstruation, you might ask, Why am I cramping my womb? This approach can help you maintain a mind-body awareness about the symptoms you experience and their connection to what you are feeling about what's going on in your life.

For instance, Camille, whose story is in chapter 2, told me that she suffered from severe headaches. Knowing that symptoms can provide valuable information about what is happening at the deepest levels of our psyches, I viewed her headache like an arrow pointing to issues that she might be either consciously or unconsciously avoiding. When I asked her, "Tell me how you are feeling when you're aching your head," Camille was taken aback. She had never thought about her headaches quite that way. My question prompted her to start taking note of when she experienced her headaches and what was occurring at the time. Camille discovered that her headaches were connected to times when she was holding in her anger—for instance, when she argued with a coworker or was stuck in traffic. These experiences reminded her of childhood incidents when she felt she could not express her feelings for fear of her mother's disapproval.

If you often have headaches or other repetitive symptoms, you may also want to start a symptom diary in your journal. By keeping a record of each symptom, what is occurring in your life at the time, and how you feel—emotionally and physically—just before and during the onset of your pain, you may see patterns emerging. Understanding what these patterns mean will help you become aware of how you live your life and how this influences your health. You can improve the quality of your life—and your reproductive health—by being aware of this important connection.

As you record your symptoms and their connections to your feelings and your life, you will see key patterns emerging that do not support your health and reproductive well-being.

For example, when you are feeling angry, do you express it—or hold it in? When you feel sad, depressed, frustrated, or like crying, what do you do with those feelings? Do you experience cold hands or feet? Contrary to popular belief, this does not mean you have a "warm heart," but rather that you are tense and your blood is not circulating as it should. Headaches are a strong indicator of rage being held in your body.

How about your lifestyle behavior? Does it include smoking, drinking, and overeating? How do you feel about this? What changes would you be willing to make? If you have physical symptoms from any of your lifestyle habits, you may be stockpiling your feelings in your body. Getting to the mind-body root of those habits and feelings is the key to improved physical health.

By applying the same process of inquiry into the health of your reproductive system, you become the designer of a uniquely exquisite and intimate language—that of your own fertility. The following process is designed to help you explore any physical symptom as a message from your body. If you are concerned about more than one symptom, continue to repeat the process so that you interpret the meaning and purpose of each message.

The five steps include:

1. Developing a physiological/medical understanding of your symptom
2. Determining how your personal history may be connected to your symptom
3. Identifying and releasing emotions you may have suppressed that contributed to your symptom
4. Treating your body as your ally
5. Tension-releasing/relaxation exercises

To illustrate how you can utilize these five steps in order to gain insight into your symptoms, I have interlaced them through the story of one client, Marie.

Step 1: Developing a Physiological/Medical Understanding of Your Physical Symptom

If you have been given a medical diagnosis, get as much factual information from your doctor as possible about your symptom. If your symptom is related to your reproductive system, it can be helpful to look at a diagram of the reproductive system for an overview of the inner structure and workings of your body. You may also want to consult a book that offers a holistic understanding of the symptom, such as Dr. Christiane Northrup's *Women's Bodies, Women's Wisdom*. Becoming an active participant in all your health-care efforts, medical and nonmedical, will increase the effectiveness of your treatments.

I have included a key visualization on page 169, "Taking Charge of Your Reproductive Procedures," which highlights the importance of this collaborative relationship.

Marie, age thirty-seven, a soap-opera writer, experienced three ectopic pregnancies. These excruciatingly painful, life-threatening pregnancies occur when an egg implants itself outside the uterus. Normally, the fimbria—the hairlike fringe at the opening of the fallopian tubes—retrieves the egg as it is released from the ovary. The egg is fertilized within the tube; then the egg divides and is carried along the tube back toward the uterus.[1] But an ectopic pregnancy can be caused by an obstruction or scarring in the fallopian tube. Additionally, when a woman feels very tense and tight, the muscles of her body, including the muscles lining her fallopian tubes, can contract and go into spasms. Instead of being open and funnel-shaped, the end of the fallopian tube may be drawn together like a duffel bag with its strings pulled tight, so that the egg becomes stuck in the tube rather than released for implantation in the uterine wall.

Step 2: Determining How Your Personal History Is Connected to Your Symptom

As we searched for emotional connections to Marie's ectopic pregnancies, I learned that one of her deeply held family secrets may have been contributing to them. At the age of fifteen, Marie's mother had become pregnant and at the same time her grandmother also became pregnant. Her mother and grandmother had left town and returned months later, with Marie's grandmother claiming she'd had twins. The truth didn't come out for another three decades. "Uncle Pete was really my brother, my mother's son. I am actually his sister," Marie said.

Family secrets can be psychologically damaging to those who hold them and to later generations from whom they are withheld. "The dark secrets that are so carefully guarded get revealed and uncovered because the children act them out—if not in this generation, then the next, or the next," writes John Bradshaw.[2] That is precisely what happened in Marie's family. Her ephistogram revealed a family pattern of babies born out of wedlock. Marie's maternal grandmother had not been married when she had Marie's mother; Marie's mother had given birth out of wedlock to her son, Peter; and Marie's three sisters had been unmarried when they each had their first children. Marie said sadly, "None of the women in my family have ever recovered from the poverty into which unwed motherhood led them." True to the family pattern, at seventeen, Marie, also unwed, had become pregnant, but she decided, "I will not live out my grandmother's, mother's, or sisters' impoverished lives." She had an abortion that she kept secret from her family because, as she said, "Mom always said I was her best daughter, and she warned me not to ruin my life with a baby. But she would have been heartbroken if she'd known about my abortion. Even after her death, I kept it a secret. I've carried this guilt for twenty years."

Even though she was taught that having a baby could ruin one's life, it was at odds with her family's code of "keep the baby no matter what." She felt tremendously guilty. "On one level, I know having an abortion was the right choice. But neither my mother nor my sisters aborted their babies. Now I have a great marriage and career that would allow me to have babies without financial ruin, but I can't have a live birth." Her pregnancies were getting stuck possibly because of the extreme tension resulting from her guilty feelings and fears.

You may have already made the connection for why a particular part of your body is being affected by your unconscious beliefs. If not, look again at the theme that your symptom is presenting. For instance, an ectopic pregnancy would have the theme of incompletion, or unwillingness to let go, or something not real or legitimate, or indecision or conflict about pregnancy.

In my work with Marie, she realized that each time she has become pregnant as a married woman, her guilt and shame for betraying her mother have been reactivated. Marie's pregnancies have become stuck in her fallopian tubes, preventing her from having a "legitimate" birth. In addition to the physical pain of her ectopic pregnancies, she suffers the emotional torment of the fertilized egg being held in her body but not becoming a baby. Marie feels as if she has been unconsciously atoning for a "sin" that she wasn't aware was so damaging to her.

The influence of your own personal history on your body can be determined by reading over your descriptions of your symptoms that you have recorded in the symptom diary in your journal. Close your eyes and sit quietly, breathe deeply, and reflect on your pain or symptom and what it might be connected to. Notice any thought or image that comes to your mind and allow yourself to see what the images represent. Write down in your journal every possible connection that comes to mind: When did you feel the symptom? What was going on in your life at the time you experienced the symptom? What were your feelings prior to its onset? If the connection between what you write and your symptom isn't immediately apparent, it may present itself to you later, sometimes in a disguised form: e.g., a song title, a magazine article.

Step 3: Identifying and Releasing Repressed Emotions That Contributed to Your Symptom

Use any of the strategies included in chapter 5 or the tension-releasing techniques at the end of this chapter to carry out this step. Pillow talk works especially well. Use the pillow to talk to that particular part of your body and then let your body talk back to you. For instance, if you have fibroids, ask the fibroids, "Why are you drawing my attention to my uterus? What wisdom do you hold for me that I have missed?"

Marie created a grief ceremony (described in chapter 5) for the babies she once carried to help her deal with her sadness. She also worked with a pillow-talk exercise, during which one of her fallopian tubes "told" her she had been carrying unjustly the emotional weight of her abortion and all the other family secrets. She said, "It's like the Christmas story, when there was no room at the inn and the baby was turned away. These family secrets are so heavy, there's no room in my uterus for a healthy pregnancy." I encouraged Marie to use the pillow-talk technique to "dialogue" with her fallopian tubes. "Symptom dialoguing" is a very effective process for asking your symptom (e.g., headache, backache, cold hands) its meaning for you, giving it a voice and trusting that what you hear in the exchange will be helpful in your healing process. Marie ultimately "made room in her uterus" for a healthy pregnancy by releasing her long-standing guilt and pain, writing long, passionate letters to her deceased mother and other members of her family (although she never mailed the letters) concerning her abortion and all she had gone through trying to conceive.

Step 4: Becoming an Ally to Your Body

This step allows you to be the most creative in utilizing your unique language of fertility. Key in this step is the healing that can occur when you no longer think of your body as an adversary, but as your ally.

Consult your inner guide for suggestions. Whatever your reproductive symptom may be, focus your energy, love, and healing light on that area of your body.

Marie developed a mantra—short phrases with positive associations and imagery—that she would repeat over and over. In the morning, at noon, and before going to bed, sometimes lying in her husband's arms, she would say to herself, "I deserve to have a healthy baby. I welcome truth, openness, and light into my body." Whenever she repeated the mantra, she visualized light filtering into her body, throughout her reproductive system, and into her fallopian tubes, untying the "knots" in her fimbria. As the light traveled on, it illuminated any dark or shadowy areas deep within her. She felt the energy move through her body. At work, over her desk, she hung a poster of one of van Gogh's sunflower paintings. The sunny, light-filled image reminded her to visualize the light illuminating the shadows of her family's secrets.

As Marie visualized her inner guide opening a book with the names of newborns, she wrote the names of her longed-for children. While riding home from work on the train, she visualized her fallopian tubes opening and working effectively. She imagined a perfect egg being released and becoming fertilized within her relaxed tube—the egg dividing, then moving along her fallopian tube toward her uterus and into her uterine cavity. Visualizations can be done anytime or anyplace and as often as possible.

Keep in mind that the language of each person's fertility is unique. However, by utilizing the process detailed above, you can at least begin to understand what meaning your ectopic pregnancy—or, for that matter, any other symptom you may be experiencing—has for you.

Step 5: Tension-Releasing/Relaxation Exercises

Thinking about your symptoms can produce anxiety. For instance, if you have miscarried and have conceived again, you may find yourself struggling with feelings of persistent anxiety, which could affect your

ability to carry your pregnancy to term (see chapter 8 for more information on miscarriages). Feeling fearful and concerned about a physical
symptom is understandable. But in the interest of healing, it is crucial
that you address the underlying issues that may be fueling your fears or
worries and keeping the symptoms going. This is of particular importance in averting miscarriages because fear and persistent anxiety can
emotionally and physically undermine a pregnancy. A child who has
been raised feeling unloved and rejected by a parent has already experienced what that child considers the worst possible loss—his mother's or
father's love—and will grow up feeling emotionally abandoned. This
can instill in him lifelong fear. If this has been your experience, the possibility of further losses, such as a miscarriage, can leave you in a constant state of panic. Anxiety is one of the factors most likely to affect
maternal-fetal bonding.[3]

You may well be thinking that anxiety isn't something that you
can control, especially if you grew up in a family of chronic worriers.
Continued healing work can help lower the level of your anxiety. The
following exercises will be very helpful in learning how to release your
negative feelings, thereby relaxing your mind-body.

EXERCISE 1: KEEPING A WORRY DIARY

One method for lowering your anxiety level is by recording your worries
in a worry diary. Keep an ongoing list of your most upsetting worries in
a small notebook. Anytime you feel yourself beginning to worry, record
in your diary the date, time, circumstances, what you were feeling, what
the worry was about, what it is connected to and what you did to seek
relief. As you fill your pages, you may want to go back through what you
have already written and underline worries that seem to be the most
persistent. One client told me that simply "bringing my worries into the
light of day, and spelling them out, took the power out of them." Carry
your diary with you wherever you go so that you can use it as often as
you need to. By recording your concerns and feelings on paper, you can

quiet negative messages in your mind. Once you've identified the underlying source of the worries, you can at some point ceremonially discard your diary.

EXERCISE 2: EXTERNALIZING AND
TRANSFERRING YOUR ANGER

If you have found that you modeled your worry style after one of your parents, the next time you feel anxious, clap your hands and say force-fully, "Mom [or Dad], get out of my head!" As Dr. Brenda Wade has said, "Hitting or stomping a surface is an important aspect of this exer-cise because it externalizes, transfers and releases the anger. Then, because our psyches never go into neutral, there must also be a positive affirmation to take the place of what was negative."

EXERCISE 3: FACING THE OLD FEARS

Review your journal and find childhood incidents that caused you to feel anxious, frightened, and unsafe. If there's more than one, try this exercise with each of the separate memories. Sit comfortably on the floor in a quiet room where you can be alone, and be mindful of the importance of continuing to breathe deeply and evenly.

Select a hurtful memory you would like to render less powerful. Imagine yourself in a protective bubble, clear but impenetrably strong. See yourself floating in that bubble back to the scene of your childhood memory. Picture the room as it was that day. Notice items in the room that are familiar. As you recall this memory, see yourself at the age you were then. How do you feel physically? What is your facial expression? If you recall coming home to an empty house at the end of a school day, for example, do you remember hearing a threatening sound? You might have felt danger was imminent. But this time, from the safety of your bubble, you call aloud to your parents. Tell them that you are afraid.

Miraculously, your parents materialize before you. Truly see them. They are here to give you what you need. See them as warm, loving, and willing to hear you. Tell them how much you needed them to protect you. Wrap your arms soothingly around your shoulders. Speak as if you were your parents, offering words of comfort. Have them reassure you and promise you that they will never leave you or let any harm befall you. Feel your sense of peace and safety. Sunlight is flooding into the room as your bubble ascends, and you look back only once, knowing with reassurance that your anxiety and fears will greatly diminish. Tell yourself that you are so loved and so worthy of happiness that you deserve peace of mind and safety. See the bubble carrying you into the present. When you alight from it, feel this sense of peace and safety throughout your mind-body.

EXERCISE 4: CHALLENGING SELF-DOUBT: LEARNING SELF-LOVE AND SELF-APPROVAL

This next exercise, which was adapted from an affirmation by mind-body pioneer Louise Hay's *You Can Heal Your Life,* can be particularly helpful when childhood experiences have instilled in you a sense of "unworthiness."

One of my clients doubted whether she would be a good mother, even though she very much wanted a baby. When she asked herself whose disapproving voice she was hearing, she was startled to hear that it was her father's. She said, "That's impossible—he's very supportive." As she continued searching for answers, however, she realized that, like many fathers, he began to pull away from her when she reached puberty, which caused her to feel anxious and rejected because she was becoming a woman. Seeing this old source of her concern, she was able to strengthen her own inner sense of herself as a woman and mother-to-be.

If you have any of these self-doubts, repeat to yourself several times a day, "I know I will be a good mother." When you say this, do you hear an inner voice saying, "No, you won't?" Do you hear any other negative responses? Stop for a moment, take a deep breath, and ask yourself whose voice(s) you hear. Record them in your journal. When these negative voices pop up, answer them from the part of you that knows in your head and heart, "I will be a good mother."

Keep repeating this exercise until you feel satisfied knowing who the "no" part of you represents and that this "no" part of you is not all of you.

Now give yourself a hug, as many times a day as possible, affirming your self-worth. If you truly want to walk the path of self-loving, take the time to listen to your heart. To live lovingly this practice is essential, because our heart is the source of our connection and intimacy with all of life—and with our fertility. Sit and listen deeply until you can hear the song of the child you hope to conceive.

EXERCISE 5: REWELCOMING YOURSELF INTO THE WORLD

Sometimes your desire to conceive may be beset by worries about yourself and the baby because your parents may not have been as loving and accepting of you as you would have liked. A woman's anxiety over a baby being born "perfect" can be an unconscious wish to be reborn as a baby her parents could fully love and accept. It may help you to resolve this need and worry by doing the following pillow-talk exercise, which will help you begin healing as you connect to your internal loving parent. I often use this exercise to allow clients to hear their ideal parent speak to them as they wished they had been spoken to in childhood and, even later, as adults.

Select a large pillow to represent your parents and another smaller pillow to represent yourself as a baby. Sitting on top of the parent pillow, speak to the pillow that represents you as a baby, saying the words you would have liked your parents to say to you. For instance, have your mother say: "I love you and I want you. You are an absolutely beautiful baby. You are perfect in every way." Then you could have your father say, "I love you and I am so proud of you." When you have finished speaking, hug the pillow that represents you and give yourself the love and approval you still crave and deserve. Accept and cherish every aspect of yourself—not only your bright and sunny disposition but also your darkest and most frightening thoughts. And then—since children love to dance—how about playing some music you love and just dance together. Great fun!

EXERCISE 6: TAKING CHARGE OF YOUR REPRODUCTIVE PROCEDURES—A GUIDED VISUALIZATION

Too often women become passive when relating to physicians, male or female, re-creating a parent-child relationship. Keep in mind that you have a right to know all the details about your treatment. You have a right to ask questions. You have a right to express your feelings when conflicted about how you were treated, such as when phone calls are not returned, and so on. "Stuffing" these feelings creates internalized tension and pressure, which, as you have learned by now, is very detrimental in general and during your fertility procedure in particular. As we noted above, it's important to be knowledgeable about the procedures, effects, and consequences of the medical fertility treatments you are undergoing. The more you know, the closer you move toward taking charge of your reproductive health.

When undergoing a procedure, consider how you are feeling emotionally and physically prior to the treatment. Suppressing your emotional reactions can work against the treatment. It is important to be in an open, relaxed, and receptive state so you can maximize the effectiveness of the process. Feeling anxious, fearful, and so on about the procedure and its outcome is perfectly understandable. It is acknowledging these emotional states that counts.

This visualization can be very helpful immediately before a medical fertility procedure. As you begin this visualization, be mindful of how you may be holding your breath to block out feelings of anxiety.

Process: Sit or stretch out in a comfortable position. Be very mindful of your breathing. Inhale deeply and exhale slowly. Know that with each inhalation you are taking into your body oxygen that cleanses and heals. With every exhalation, know you are eliminating toxins from your body. Continuing to focus on your breathing, allow yourself to become aware of any areas of tension from the top of your head throughout your body. With each breath, inhale more deeply, and as you exhale, send your breath down to your uterus, ovaries, cervix, fallopian tubes, and vagina. Visualize your whole reproductive system pulsating with the energy of your breath. As you deepen your breathing, exhale slowly, releasing any tension you may be feeling in these areas. As you grow increasingly calm, visualize a warm, gentle, slow current, like a warm liquid, flowing from the base of your skull downward in a circular caressing motion to all parts of your body, inside and out, down to the very tips of your toes. Take a deep breath and release. Continue to see yourself feeling warm and relaxed. When you sense any tension or anxiety arising, breathe into it and release the tension. If there still is any additional tension remaining in your body, see yourself rolling it up in a ball and disposing of it. What's most important is that you stay connected with what you are truly feeling while you are undergoing a procedure, even in your process of relaxing. Take several long stretches, slowly bringing your consciousness back into the room, opening your eyes, and feeling refreshed and more centered.

If you are crying or feel like crying, feel free to do so. Own your space and your feelings. With your body and mind in harmony, any tension that is present becomes considerably lessened. As your body opens to accept new life, the chances for a successful procedure are greatly increased.

Use the five-step program at the beginning of this chapter as you explore each of your symptoms. In the next few chapters, we will focus on three major reproductive difficulties that many women face. The tension-releasing/relaxation techniques discussed in Step 5 can be used as needed while you read through the rest of Part Three and whenever you feel it is necessary.

SEVEN

Menstrual and Ovulation Irregularities

As women, our menstrual cycles are part of our inner guidance system, which "is the most basic, earthy cycle we have."[1] It signals the most important transition in our lives, from childhood to womanhood. Our menstrual cycle, the most sensitive part of ourselves, responds to conflicted feelings powerful enough to block a pregnancy.

If you have been diagnosed with a menstrual or ovulation irregularity, think of your symptom as a beacon of light in the darkness, lighting the way for you to draw the powers of your mind to the area of your body where your energy is blocked. The first step in creating a healthier environment for your menstrual cycle is to develop an understanding of how it works and what can interfere with its healthy functioning.

Just for a moment, picture an orchestra with its dozens of instruments, each playing a part in a symphonic score. Now visualize the synchronized interaction of your brain, limbic system, hypothalamus, pituitary, ovaries, and hormonal secretions—which culminate in the maturation and release of a fertilized egg, or, when pregnancy doesn't occur, the cyclical shedding of your endometrium. Remember that, like the musical instruments, which are guided by the mind and heart of a conductor in an orchestra, the parts of your reproductive system work together harmoniously or disharmoniously as a result of the conscious and unconscious messages that you send as the conductor of your body and life. These messages either promote or interrupt the harmonious functioning of your menstrual cycle.

As you read this chapter, if you have experienced any disruption of your menstrual cycle, keep in mind the five-step program described in the previous chapter as well as these steps:

1. Recall what was occurring in your life when you began to experience menstrual irregularities. Ask yourself what feelings were evoked.

2. Explore your childhood experiences for a theme or series of experiences connected to these present-day emotions.

3. Look closely at your first menses for more clues to your beliefs about menstruation and pregnancy.

4. Consider what your symptoms may be trying to tell you about what's going on in your life concerning conception.

When a young woman's brain signals her hypothalamus to release gonadotropin-releasing hormone (GnRH) every hour and a half, twenty-four hours a day, her ovaries and pituitary react by releasing other hormones, and her first menses begins. It often takes another two or three years for her ovaries to begin releasing eggs regularly every month, which usually begins when she is about fourteen or fifteen. This process is set off by GnRH, which travels from the hypothalamus through tiny blood vessels to the pituitary, which then secretes quantities of follicle-stimulating hormone (FSH). FSH stimulates the growth of fluid-filled cavities called follicles. Receptors on the estrogen-producing cells of the ovaries absorb FSH. The pituitary also secretes smaller amounts of luteinizing hormone (LH).

Inside the ovaries, in response to higher FSH levels, eggs (ova) begin to develop. The first fluid-filled follicle to become the largest grows close to the ovary's outer surface. In response to increasing levels of estrogen, the pituitary slows FSH production.[2]

The ovulation process is timed to work with the monthly changes in the uterine lining's endometrial cells. Each month, the uterine lining reddens and grows spongy, preparing to provide a nourishing bed for an egg cell should fertilization occur. When estrogen has been maintained at peak levels for forty-eight hours, the hypothalamus steps up secretion of GnRH, which triggers the pituitary to send more LH. "When the LH surge has been maintained for about twenty-four hours, the wall of the follicle disintegrates and the surface ruptures," writes Carla Harkness. "The miracle of ovulation occurs as a fertile ovum, only ⅟₅₀ inch in diameter, is released from the ovary."[3] When fertilization does not occur, the uterine lining is shed through the vagina as the menstrual flow begins again.

The period of ten to fourteen days between the time a woman ovulates and before she begins menstruating is referred to as the luteal phase of a woman's cycle. But when the phase lasts nine days or less, or when the level of progesterone secreted is too low, the woman is considered to have a luteal-phase defect. According to Carla Harkness, this problem, which occurs in about 5 percent of patients struggling with reproductive problems, prevents women from achieving or sustaining pregnancy, and they often miscarry. A low level of progesterone may be responsible for "…an inadequate maturation of the endometrial lining. The embryo then has difficulty implanting and surviving its early gestation."[4]

Amenorrhea

With ovulation and menstruation regulated by hormonal secretions, these processes are, of course, affected by our emotional states. In situations of extreme tension, many women do not ovulate and stop menstruating. When a woman stops having her period, this condition is sometimes referred to as hypothalamic amenorrhea. From my perspective, amenorrhea in a woman who wants to conceive is often the mind-body's way of revealing the intense conflict around being pregnant.

My experiences have been borne out by the ongoing research concerning women diagnosed with hypothalamic amenorrhea that was conducted by Sarah L. Berga, M.D., at Magee Women's Hospital, Pittsburgh, Pennsylvania. She concluded that emotional tension is one of the major factors effecting a decline in the hypothalamic secretion of GnRH, reducing the pituitary secretion of LH and FSH, which leads to insufficient ovarian stimulation to support menstruation.

If you were diagnosed as having amenorrhea, your awareness of its connection to what is going on in your life now as well as knowledge of your family history will help you understand what your body is trying to tell you. Some of my clients say, "I feel too tired to become a mother," "I'm too sad" ("too inferior," "too empty"), or "I'm so afraid I will do to my children what my mother did to me." One of the messages that many of my clients eventually receive from their bodies concerning their irregular menstrual functioning is this: I'm too frightened to become a mother. The two clients' stories that follow can help you explore any issues you may have concerning your menstrual cycle.

One woman whose childhood experiences had left her quite fearful was Ann, a forty-year-old chef at one of Manhattan's trendiest restaurants. She said during our first session that her period had stopped one year before. Her doctor was unable to offer medical explanations for her amenorrhea and predicted that her period would never resume. Ann and her husband, Klaus, age thirty-nine, a photographer, told me, "We've been thinking about having a baby." Ann added, "We've had our eye on my biological clock." Ann's mother had started menopause at forty, so Ann feared that she already was menopausal.

Although many people are unable to remember what they were experiencing around the time they stopped menstruating, Ann said she would never forget. The week before Ann stopped menstruating, her neighbor had been involved in a brutal carjacking, and a week later, when Ann returned from work, some teenagers rear-ended her and chased after her in their car. When she drove to the parking lot of a busy supermarket and screamed for help, the boys sped off. After hearing her description of her pursuers, police confirmed that they were the same boys who had attacked her neighbor. "I've never driven by myself at night again, but I've been terrified that somehow they'd find out where I live and finish what they'd started. Unfortunately, since the night of that incident, I've never gotten my period again."

While I could certainly understand the tremendous fear an event like this could engender for Ann, I sensed that for it to have had such a profound effect on her physiologically, it may have triggered feelings she had repressed concerning a traumatic childhood experience that had made her feel threatened and unsafe.

If you have some recollection of the time when you stopped menstruating, consider whatever was occurring in your life during that time as the tip of the iceberg and check to see if this incident is somehow connected to an earlier experience. For example, you may have stopped menstruating during a time when you felt unsafe, unsupported, or rejected. If so, try to connect those events to experiences during your childhood, particularly those surrounding your first period, when you had no power to take control of your own life.

By writing in her journal about her first menstruation, Ann found the first of many vital clues that would lead to understanding the cessation of menses later in life. "My mother said my period was something terrible that women had to bear, and she treated it like a deep, dark, dirty secret and hid our sanitary napkins and belts in the linen closet. Each month, I was deathly afraid of my father or brother knowing when I had my period."

Like Ann, many women have had negative initial experiences with their first menses. Clients have shared numerous stories about how they were made to feel frightened and shameful about their natural female cycles and taught that their periods were "the curse." One woman's mother told her not to touch plants when she was menstruating, because she could kill them. Another said, "My mother warned that this was a terrible thing for a woman to endure and that I would suffer from excruciating cramps and be bedridden."

In many ancient cultures, a woman's first period is welcomed with tribal rituals. Women's cycles are considered the human embodiment of larger cosmic cycles, especially those of the moon. In our culture, however, women have been discouraged from trusting their body's natural energy flow. Patriarchal teachings and attitudes over generations have cloaked this natural process in taboos and distortions.

In Ann's situation, the secrecy surrounding her period pointed to an overarching family theme of fear, shame, and secrets. One of her parents' most closely guarded secrets was that they were first cousins. It is reported that first cousins have a high chance of sharing recessive traits that could be lethal to one in four of their offspring. As her parents' first child, Ann absorbed her mother's shame, guilt, and fear surrounding her birth. Although Ann was born healthy, her mother continued to act out of fear, fighting Ann's attempts to become autonomous, rewarding her when she acted needy and helpless. Ann's mother needed her to be dependent on her and infantile, and so she treated Ann's menses as an unwanted sign she was a woman.

When Ann was seven, her sister was born. Her sister was quite sickly for the first year of her life, confirming her mother's greatest fears of the "first cousins' marriage curse." With her mother spending most of her days at the hospital, tending to her infant, Ann was left with neighbors, where, she said, "I felt completely abandoned."

As Ann reviewed her past, she discovered that she has always felt unsafe because her parents, who had been political prisoners in a Latin American country, had fled illegally to the United States and lived in constant fear of deportation. "I felt I could never really be safe, and that the government would take us away." Her terrifying confrontation with the carjackers had triggered her internalized parents' terror as well as reawakened her early-childhood fears and her tremendous need to feel safe and protected by her mother and, now, her husband.

Ann eventually identified the messages being sent to her by her not menstruating. She was feeling a lack of safety and was fearful of being a woman. She realized that when she reached puberty, she had felt the need to hide her growing breasts and any other sign of womanliness from her mother. "I don't know why, but for some reason, I believed that if I wasn't a child, she couldn't protect me anymore."

To help Ann resolve and release these feelings, I encouraged her to do a pillow-talk exercise. Ann set up a "mother" pillow, and when she began to cry, she said through tears. "I'm afraid of getting pregnant and not being your little girl anymore. You won't love and protect me and I'll be abandoned again, the way you left me when my sister was born."

As Ann continued speaking, she suddenly began coughing uncontrollably. Ann had written on her profile that her mother had suffered from a hacking cough throughout her pregnancy with Ann. When Ann's coughing subsided long enough for her to continue talking, she told her "mother" pillow, "I felt you didn't want me because you were so frightened I'd be deformed, and that you were trying to cough me up, get me out from inside you. And that's what I know I now need to do to you—get you and your fears out of my head." For the first time, she was able to release the anger she felt toward her mother for abandoning her and fostering such dependency and fear in her.

Ann had resisted telling her mother about her menstrual irregularities, though I had encouraged her to do so. At this point in our work, Ann said, "I feel stronger now, not so frightened. I'm going to talk to my mother tonight." This would be the first signal in their relationship that Ann was no longer willing to remain in a dependent, childlike state. That night, in addition to discussing her reproductive problems, she also told her mother she planned to adopt if she was unable to conceive. It was the first time she had said these words aloud. Ann had been keeping her adoption plans a secret, even from herself. Her first step toward openness and emotional adulthood paid off. "The next morning, I woke up with cramps, and then my period started," Ann said, sounding astonished. She added, "It's a full, regular period."

Her monthly cycles have been regular and Ann has continued to work on separating emotionally from her mother. The house Ann and her husband had been living in was dark and on a noisy street. They have recently moved to a safe neighborhood and have purchased a new home—this one is sun-filled, with lots of open spaces and a room for a nursery. The house is symbolic of Ann's new life—out of the darkness, into the light of understanding.

Dysfunctional Uterine Bleeding

About one-third of the women who begin working with me for menstrual irregularities experience extremely heavy menstrual bleeding. If this is a problem for you, you may also want to take time to consider how this symptom fits into your family history. Ask your body what this symptom is trying to tell you and how it has affected your life.

Evelyn, a twenty-four-year-old model, was bleeding excessively because of severe fibroid tumors. The tumors had grown in her uterine wall and her doctor had advised that if the bleeding couldn't be controlled, Evelyn would have to have a hysterectomy. She was frightened about her impending surgery, which had been scheduled for two months from the date of our first session.

When I asked Evelyn when her excessive bleeding began, she said, "Soon after I accepted my boyfriend's marriage proposal." As I have noted before, questioning your body to determine what your symptom is trying to tell you is most important in order to ultimately trigger your healing process. Evelyn continued, "I felt that getting married would mean having children. Before that, I never had any desire to become a mother, and I didn't have any problems with my menstrual cycle. But in the last six months, I've actually been contemplating pregnancy. Now I don't know if I can become pregnant."

Evelyn's family history and sibling relationships revealed several key connections. She is the eldest of five sisters and two brothers, and her parents, who were preoccupied with building a car dealership, she said, "bullied me into taking care of the kids." Since she was only ten months older than the brother closest to her age, her duties as a substitute mother began as far back as she could recall. "I diapered my sisters and brothers, prepared their bottles, fed them, and later I cleaned up after them, washed their clothes, and cooked for them."

I asked her to draw her siblings, and when she had finished, she gasped when she realized she had sketched a bird's nest with seven siblings looking up at her. "Oh my God, they look like seven gaping mouths waiting to be fed—by me." She began crying as she said, "Experiencing all these responsibilities day by day was one thing, but when I see how many children I've mothered, it takes my breath away. That's why I never wanted to have children before. And judging from my bleeding, I'm afraid I don't really want them now."

At the age of eleven, Evelyn began menstruating. Although her mother had never prepared her for it, Evelyn sensed it had something to do with pregnancy, because she had seen her mother pregnant year after year. When she started menstruating, her mother said, "This blood is a sign that you are a woman now. You've got to be careful or you could get pregnant." It is rather sad how few women experienced this important rite of passage in a positive, wondrous way. Rather, with the first sign of menstrual bleeding, most women, like Evelyn, were made to feel fearful about entering puberty.

Her mother's warning that she could get pregnant is one that has been repeated in households the world over. While it is typically offered to be helpful, it can be a powerful and potentially damaging message if you were made to feel, along with other childhood events, that your life could be ruined by motherhood. Years later, when Evelyn wanted to become a mother, her body became the messenger of her unconscious fears. As long as she was bleeding heavily, pregnancy was out of the question.

We worked together for two months, releasing the anger and sadness she felt about having been a substitute mother so young, when Evelyn experienced a breakthrough. Her heavy menstrual bleeding finally had stopped. Her doctors canceled the surgery to have her fibroids and possibly her uterus removed.

There are many things you can do to take action in your life to strengthen your view of yourself as a healthy, fertile woman. Start by asking your inner guide for direction. Communicate directly with your mind-body by assuring yourself that you are strong and womanly and welcome either a return of your menstrual cycle or cessation of undue menstrual bleeding. It is crucial that you remain patient and loving with your body.

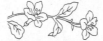

SELF-EXPLORATION

To explore the beliefs you developed in childhood in response to your family situation, try utilizing the pillow-talk exercise in chapter 5. Tell your mother or your father why you felt so frightened, or insecure, or angry, or sad, for instance, that you could not allow yourself to have your period and feel like a woman—possibly a pregnant woman. Try beginning your sentences with "I feel [fill in the word] and that's why I can't have my period." You might want to tape-record what you have to say, or, soon afterward, write down what you have said. The answer to your conflict lies in your mind-body communication system and the extent to which you have held back all your unexpressed feelings. You will probably have a lot to say now.

In keeping with the harmonious working of your body, you may want to begin your day by playing a selection of your favorite soothing music. As you listen, close your eyes, breathe deeply, and visualize the smooth functioning of your menstrual cycle.

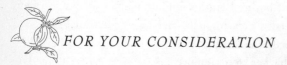 *FOR YOUR CONSIDERATION*

Can you recall your initial reaction to your first menstrual cycle? Was it positive or negative? Why? If there was an air of secrecy and shame in your home concerning your period, how do you think that affected you? Was this feeling of secrecy or shame—or any conflicted emotion surrounding your period—an overarching theme in your childhood?

How old were your mother and the other women in your family when they went through menopause? If you are over forty, are you concerned that irregularities in your menstrual cycle are connected to menopause? Take some time to recall the details of what was happening in your life when your period became irregular.

EIGHT

Miscarriages: "How Can I Hold My Pregnancy to Term?"

 Pregnancy is a joyous state of being, but for women who miscarry, a lost pregnancy can cause intense pain, anguish, and grief. If you have experienced a miscarriage or are worried about having one, this chapter will comfort you and open new possibilities for you to carry your pregnancy to term. In working with clients who have experienced these losses, I have found that exploring emotionally based issues—from childhood conflicts to ambivalence about motherhood—can prevent recurrence of miscarriages. A growing number of health-care professionals agree.

Dinora Pines, a London-based therapist, concludes from her work with women who have miscarried that conflicts belonging to past developmental stages in childhood be explored particularly before or during a first pregnancy. Pines states, "Where ambivalent feelings toward the mother have been unresolved, or where negative feelings towards the self, the sexual partner or important figures from the past predominate…pregnancy facilitates the projection of such feelings onto the fetus.…The fetus may be physically retained, given life and cocooned or may be physically rejected as in miscarriage and abortion. If the patient is in analysis during pregnancy, analysis of her conflicts may in some cases lead to a successful pregnancy and to the birth of a baby."[1]

This certainly has been the experience of a considerable number of my clients.

Making this connection to past experiences and feelings is not about placing blame for a miscarriage. When you are in pain, it's almost instinctual to blame someone—even yourself—but as we have discussed all through this process, blaming is harmful to your health. It can take away your energy and focus from healing and cause you to feel like a victim. As my clients begin to liberate themselves from blame and explore the life events—past and present—surrounding their miscarriages, most have been able to carry their next pregnancies to term.

Similar outcomes were found by R. L. Vandenbergh in a study of women who had experienced recurring miscarriages. Several of the women in the study who worked with therapists and learned how to express their anger directly rather than to contain it in their bodies had a success rate of 80 percent for maintaining subsequent pregnancies. Among those women who did not enter into therapy, the success rate was only 6 percent.[2]

These results certainly suggest that your emotional state can determine your receptivity to conception and whether or not your embryo implants itself so you can carry your pregnancy to term. As we have discussed in previous chapters, conflicting messages can signal your body to reject a pregnancy, despite your conscious longing and love for your unborn child.

An estimated one in four women has experienced a miscarriage and one in three hundred has had three or more miscarriages in a row.[3] Dr. Jonathan Scher, a pioneer in the field of miscarriage prevention, believes that scientists only now are realizing the high frequency of miscarriages, because modern early pregnancy tests can quickly diagnose conception. Dr. Scher writes, "In general, we can now accept that from 50 to 60 percent of first pregnancies miscarry, and that figure may in reality be higher.... As many as 75 percent of all fertilized eggs, including those that never implant, do not yield a full-term baby." Dr. Scher adds, "Of diagnosed pregnancies, however, where the woman knows she is pregnant, the rate is reassuringly lower—about 10 to 20 percent will end in miscarriage."[4]

In a majority of cases, miscarriages are not solely biological events that just happen without a reason. Researchers Robert J. Weil, M.D., and C. Tupper write, "The pregnant woman functions as a communications system. The fetus is a source of continuous messages to which the mother responds with subtle psychobiological adjustments. Her personality, influenced by her ever-changing life situation, can either act upon the fetus to maintain its constant growth and development or create physiological changes that can result in [miscarriages]. The ways in which a woman's body modulates her feelings about her pregnancy are diverse, but all are mediated by the immune and endocrine systems."[5] Since this communications system is affected by a woman's emotional state, unconscious messages from her storehouse of painful childhood memories can be transmitted to her immune and endocrine systems and contribute to a miscarriage.

To understand how your immune system can govern your pregnancy, it's important to understand how this system works. The immune system is comprised of cells that move through the bloodstream to defend us against any substance that is considered foreign to our body, such as bacteria or viruses. When the immune system is working properly, it defends against foreign invaders by producing antibodies (chemical substances produced by cells) or by the stimulation of specialized cells, which can destroy an invading organism or neutralize its toxic effects.[6]

The immune system's vigilance is not always welcome when it pertains to pregnancy. Since a developing embryo bears both the father's and the mother's molecular signature, ordinarily your body would recognize this combination as foreign and your immune system would manufacture antibodies to destroy it. "To keep this from happening," explains Dr. Niels Lauersen, "nature has provided you with an automatic protective biological response to pregnancy—blocking antibodies. They keep your body from attacking your baby. You begin to manufacture them the moment you become pregnant."[7]

In an estimated 30 percent of recurring miscarriages, however, the immune system remains on alert, blocking antibodies are suppressed, and the mother miscarries.[8] This is one of many known organic causes of miscarriages. In one study, researchers also found that the immune systems of some women produce "a suspected embryo killer called APA (antiphospholipid antibody)."[9]

What would cause a woman's immune system to attack her embryo? From my perspective, when we don't recognize our ambivalence about the pregnancy and what it is connected to, and are not aware of feeling angry, anxious, or fearful, these emotional states are communicated via the hypothalamus's neurotransmitted messages to the immune system to treat the fetus as a hostile invader. Dr. Northrup writes that hormones are "messenger molecules for emotions and thoughts. The immune cells, too, have receptors for neuropeptides [which work in a manner similar to hormones]. . . . Ovaries and probably the uterus make estrogen and progesterone—hormones that are also neurotransmitters that affect emotions and thoughts. And these organs, too, have receptor sites that receive messages from the brain and the immune system."[10]

As you read about the direct communication that occurs between your thoughts and emotions and your immune and endocrine systems, be aware of any self-blaming messages that may come into your consciousness. Write them down in your journal to use them for a visualization described later in this chapter.

Considering our mind-body communications network, it's understandable that conflicted emotions and thoughts can disrupt the synchronization of the endocrine system, which releases hormones into the bloodstream. One indication of the emotional connection in miscarriages is a finding made by British researchers; it indicates that LH, the hormone responsible for ovulation, may be connected to miscarriages. The study focused on 193 women who were planning to conceive. "After testing it was found that those women who had an elevated serum LH level prior to getting pregnant (tested on the seventh day of their menstrual cycles), had a miscarriage rate of 65 percent, as compared with 12 percent of those who had a normal LH reading," explains Dr. Niels Lauersen.[11]

The study can best be understood when you consider that the pituitary is an endocrine gland that produces LH. As you may recall, the hypothalamus is also the relay station for transmitting conscious and unconscious emotionally induced messages to our reproductive organs and directs hormonal activities via the pituitary. Another hormonal imbalance connected to miscarriages is known as the luteal-phase defect—discussed in the previous chapter—in which a woman's body does not produce sufficient levels of the hormone progesterone to sustain her pregnancy.[12] Both luteal-phase defect and elevated LH levels are reminders that we must address the emotional as well as the physical content of our lives. Our cells contain our unconscious memories, of which our conscious mind may be completely unaware. I'm not suggesting that we are at the mercy of our unconscious mind, but I do believe we can affect negatively even the most minute facets of our biochemistry and physiology.

My work with Tamra, a thirty-eight-year-old municipal court judge in Connecticut, and her husband, Bruce, age thirty-seven, a librarian, underscores the significance of addressing the interplay between negative childhood experiences and miscarriages. The couple had been living together for twelve years, had been married for six, and had been trying to conceive for eighteen months before they came to me for an initial consultation. Bruce had been diagnosed as having a low sperm count. Throughout our work together, Tamra, who had never been pregnant, took the fertility drug Pergonal, as prescribed by her physician. The year before, she'd undergone a hysterosalpingogram, and her doctor advised her that she had a T-shaped uterus, meaning that if she conceived, she might be at risk for a miscarriage or premature labor because her cervix might not be able to support a growing baby. This condition generally is found in women whose mothers used the synthetic hormone diethylstilbestrol (DES). Tamra's mother had not been given the drug, so the doctor's diagnosis of a T-shaped uterus remained puzzling and ominous.

In an effort to allay Tamra's fear and anxiety fueled by the medical diagnosis, I related the experience of Kenna, whose mother was given DES. Kenna had received very similar warnings about her uterus. Although an irregularly shaped uterus possibly can cause medical complications, in my experience it seemed only one of several factors that could have been blocking Kenna, who had three or more miscarriages, from holding a pregnancy to term.

After we engaged in working through her issues with her mother, husband, and adopted four-year-old son, Kenna did conceive, went full term, and had a daughter, Angelica. This story helped Tamra to feel considerably more relieved and less anxious as we continued to explore her core issues affecting her ability to hold her pregnancy.

As a substitute teacher, Bruce earned far less than Tamra. During the course of our first month's work, this was one of the many issues we touched upon. Tamra was fearful of living on Bruce's part-time income. Like Tamra, many working women who are major breadwinners fear becoming economically dependent on their husbands because they are not secure in the fact that their husbands will be able to provide for them and the baby, especially if they have to take extended or unpaid maternity leaves. Addressing Tamra's concerns about his lack of profes-sional ambition, Bruce tried to understand why he lacked motivation. He admitted that he worried about having a baby because, he said, "the world is such a hostile and dangerous place that it's difficult to keep a child safe from harm."

It became apparent that it was Bruce who felt his safety was threat-ened, not Tamra. He explained that when he was four, his mother had thrown his alcoholic father out of the house. Bruce had not seen his father in thirty-three years. In our work together, Bruce began to acknowledge the anger and fear he had developed in response to feel-ing utterly alone in childhood, without his father's love and support.

As a consequence of our exploration and his emotional-release work, Bruce's view of himself as "not much of a man" began to shift. He eventually reconciled with his father, visited him in Chicago, and established a relationship. After a month of intensive work, Tamra con-ceived. A month later, they opted to discontinue their therapy, despite my strong recommendation to the contrary. Her mother had convinced her that Tamra would hurt her baby by "dwelling on negative thoughts," in spite of my assurance that our bodies remain healthy when our feelings are expressed, not repressed. But Tamra insisted on "not taking any chances with the baby."

Many people believe that pregnant women need to surround themselves with only "good" thoughts. You may have received similar advice during a pregnancy. In the past, many psychologists also supported this position. "One of the most peculiar myths among some psychoanalysts of the past generation was that when a woman in analysis became pregnant, the analysis might as well cease," writes Ernest Rossi, Ph.D. "It was believed that during pregnancy women would take an artificial 'flight into health,' and so be resistant to the hard work of undoing psychodynamic repressions." On the contrary, Rossi believes that what is true is that "hormonal shifts" render a pregnant woman "open and available to personality change and transformation," and, further, that psychological support during pregnancy offers opportunities for growth and personal transformation.[13]

I told Tamra and Bruce, "Our work together is also about creating the integrity of life in your womb by being completely honest with your unborn child." But the goal-oriented Tamra felt that since conception had been achieved, our work was done, despite her worries about having a miscarriage.

First-Trimester Miscarriages—The Silent Loss

Unfortunately, Tamra did miscarry, and she got back in touch with me. Most of my clients who have had miscarriages have had them early in their pregnancies. Studies indicate that the majority of miscarriages do occur in the first trimester (weeks one through twelve) of pregnancy, which, sadly, is what happened to Tamra and Bruce.[14] Tamra sobbed as she explained that she'd miscarried in her fourth week. "I was in for a sonogram and the technician was getting a very faint heartbeat. I read on this woman's face what she was afraid to tell me: that my baby was going to die; that in the next couple of days, I'd have a miscarriage." A few days afterward, the baby died. The most painful calls I receive are those from women like Tamra, who have either recently miscarried or who have faced this loss in the past. When Bruce joined us on the phone and I asked him how he felt about the loss, he said, "Tamra's pregnancy wasn't as much a reality for me yet. She hadn't wanted me to tell anyone, but I've told people in my family."

Like many men whose wives miscarry, Bruce believed he had to keep up a "brave, manly" front; therefore, he suppressed his own feelings. I have heard men say that they couldn't allow themselves to cry over their pregnancy loss. Bruce said, "One of us has to be strong. I have to take care of my wife." Others want to be sympathetic with their wives but cannot understand the degree of their wives' devastation over losing a fetus during its early gestation.

Like Tamra, if you experienced a miscarriage, you may have been surprised by the enormity of your grief, especially because you had almost no time to prepare for the loss. Like millions of other women, Tamra, from the earliest stages of pregnancy, recognized her developing fetus as an integral part of herself.[15] Researchers L. G. Peppers and R. J. Knapp found no differences in the intensity or patterns of grief among women who experienced a spontaneous abortion (the clinical term for miscarriage), stillbirth, or neonatal death.

Your loss may have felt so painful because there is almost an immediate physiological bonding between a mother and her fetus. "The major changes in a woman's hormonal makeup take place *early* in pregnancy, almost just after conception," writes Jonathan Scher, M.D. "Mothers undergo huge hormonal fluctuations, and we tend to think this grows along with her swelling belly. But, in fact, the greatest impact of maternal feeling occurs *early* in the pregnancy. So, when you lose a pregnancy, it does feel just like you have lost a child, an anticipated child. There is scientific (hormonal) proof that these feelings occur!"[16]

The Importance of Bereavement After a Miscarriage

In an attempt to avoid pain, many women struggle to avoid grieving over a miscarriage, but it is vital for emotional recovery and growth to mourn fully such profound losses. Dr. Charles L. Whitfield writes that grief can manifest itself in "chronic anxiety, tension, fear or nervousness, anger or resentment, sadness, emptiness, unfulfillment, confusion, guilt, shame, or, as is common among many who grew up in a troubled family, as feelings of numbness or 'no feelings at all.' "[17] It's important to grieve because, as Whitfield writes, "When we allow ourselves to *feel* these painful feelings, and when we share the grief with safe, supportive, and loving others, we are able to complete our grief work and thus be free of it."[18]

If you have miscarried, even if it was early on, it is a big deal, and it needs to be treated with the respect you and your unborn baby deserve. Some professionals advocate avoiding baby showers after a miscarriage because social events such as these stimulate painful feelings. You may want to avoid any such events immediately after your miscarriage, as it is of utmost importance to be especially kind and nurturing toward yourself after such a loss. But avoiding baby showers and similar celebratory events like children's birthdays, as well as staying away from pregnant friends or relatives, sends a "closed-down," fear-based message to your reproductive system. It's important to open yourself to all of your painful feelings, allowing yourself to move back into life—all of life. Accepting yourself and all of your experiences and feelings—sadness as well as joy—creates a more receptive place within, a place in which you can be open to conceive again.

As you may have already discovered, grief is not something we can ever escape. Among women who do not mourn, symptoms of grief have been observed twenty years after their miscarriages.[19] You may find that a current loss can remind you of prior ungrieved losses that have been stored in your unconscious emotional memory bank, which has no sense of time.

In a Columbia University study (conducted from 1981 to 1982) of twenty-two women who experienced miscarriages, researchers found that "guilt was the state that appeared to be the most difficult for women and their spouses to resolve without help."[20] I have heard women worry that they miscarried for reasons that included attending a friend's wedding, picking strawberries, or taking a walk. Of course, none of these activities is enough to cause a woman to miscarry a healthy pregnancy.

But these normally logical women are in so much pain and so desperate to find an answer as to why they haven't carried their pregnancies to term, they blame themselves.

I have also observed a pattern of self-blame connected to the genetic testing generally administered to women over thirty-five during the sixteenth week of pregnancy. The results often affect a woman's decision about whether or not to maintain or clinically abort her fetus. Responding to this fear, many women consciously withhold from emotionally bonding with their babies in order to protect themselves from emotional pain should they decide they have to abort. This is unfortunate, for there is scientific validation in the latest research of prenatal bonding that confirms the importance of acknowledging the fetus at the moment of conception.

Typical of many, one young woman I met said of her first months of pregnancy, "I don't want to even think about being pregnant until I'm sure the baby's okay." Her attitude was consistent with results indicating that even women with planned pregnancies who are scheduled to undergo prenatal testing are reluctant to become "involved" with their babies until they are proven "normal."[21] Since the mind and the body are interconnected, emotional detachment can also mean not "attaching" physically.

Despite their early maternal feelings, some women tell me that if they get pregnant again, they won't tell anyone but their husbands. Francine, who is forty-one, experienced three miscarriages before working with me. She said, "The next time, I'll only tell people when I know the baby is all right. If I had another miscarriage, I couldn't stand to see the disappointment everyone feels for me."

I counseled Francine against closing herself off this way, because I generally advocate that from the moment you feel you are pregnant, or your pregnancy is confirmed, you allow yourself to open joyfully to the experience. Keeping a pregnancy secret sets into motion an energy system that makes your condition feel not quite real. By publicly declaring the news, you can strengthen your pregnancy by sending a positive emotional message to your fetus: Welcome, baby. I am so glad you are here. My intention is to carry you to term. No other moment in your pregnancy equals the joy of when you first discover you're pregnant. No matter what else is occurring in your life, or what may happen later on, it's awe-inspiring to realize you're carrying a new life inside you.

In addition to self-blame, many women who miscarry often blame their health practitioners. After Ethel, a thirty-three-year-old police detective, miscarried in her thirteenth week of pregnancy—just as her mother had miscarried during her thirteenth week, when Ethel was two years old—she was furious with her doctor. "I wanted her to keep me and my baby from harm," Ethel said. Her physician asked Ethel to bring in her fetus so they could look for clues to the miscarriage. Ethel said, "I put the baby in a plastic bag and swung the bag over the office counter, telling the receptionist I'd brought my son in for a checkup," Ethel said. "I knew that this was not a normal thing to do when I saw the look in the receptionist's eyes, as if she was thinking, Oh, dear, let me get the doctor, quick!"

Interestingly enough, Ethel's visit to the doctor was an important step in her grieving process. "I thought looking at my baby would be horrible," Ethel said, "but it wasn't. I'm so glad I saw him before I buried him, or I would always have wondered." Her physician understood that respecting Ethel's connection to her fetus could add to a sense of closure, rather than leave her unconsciously imagining the worst or becoming mired in anger, guilt, or despair.

Freeing ourselves of these negative feelings is also important because when such feelings remain in your mind-body, they can be powerful enough to contribute to further reproductive problems. In a study of 195 couples with a history of recurring miscarriages, researchers B. Stray-Pedersen and S. Stray-Pedersen noted that among women who were involved in recovery programs that offered emotional support, 85 percent of the women conceived again, while of the women in the control group who had not been given psychological support, only 35 percent had successful pregnancies.[22] Women who have not allowed themselves to mourn their losses have told me that their unresolved grief diminished the level of joy they might have experienced in their current pregnancies. If you feel you have not fully grieved over a miscarriage, I recommend that you express what you are feeling—verbally or nonverbally—by engaging in some form of grief ceremony and writing a letter to your unborn child, instructions for which can be found in chapter 5.

Tamra and Bruce tearfully participated in a grief ceremony for their lost child. She began by saying to her unborn child, "Travel on. Perhaps you will wait in the wings until I'm stronger. Maybe the next time you'll come through all the way and this will not be a doll I'm holding." She held the doll skyward. "Godspeed you on your journey. May this release create a space in me for this to happen again." And we all three said, "Amen."

Weeks after Tamra and Bruce's grief ceremony, she said she felt a sense of peace, and she began working with her doctors again, continuing her cycles of Pergonal. Twice a day, Tamra practiced the fertility visualization described on pages 169–170. To our great delight, a month after we had begun working together again, Tamra conceived. This time, although she was determined to remain in my fertility program, she found that her reproductive health was being undermined by her tremendous fear that she might miscarry again. Tamra, realizing that fleeing from negative thoughts had not protected her first pregnancy, now was willing to look at her difficult relationships with her mother and sister, and to examine the internalized parental voices and fears affecting her. Tamra's mother, a popular debutante, had been raised by a nanny in a wealthy household. Her mother and father, rarely home, lived their lives outside the home. Tamra's mother repeated the same pattern in her marriage, with Tamra being raised by a nanny. Tamra tearfully stated that "my mother didn't like babies. Even as a small child, I have no memory of spending any time at all with my mother. Nannies cared for me. My mother didn't even have friends who had babies. I used to beg her for baby dolls, but all I got were Barbie dolls, which is exactly the way my mother and my sister saw themselves."

Tamra's older sister, Grace, emphatically declared that she was never going to have children—and didn't. As Tamra became more aware of the painful baggage she was carrying around, she allowed herself to release years of buried anger and pain at never having been lovingly mothered. She also saw that her sister was caught up in their mother's negativity toward having children. Tamra developed a personalized mantra, "I'm in charge of my life now and I am creating a life for me and my baby that is safe and secure."

As Tamra continued to progress in her pregnancy and in our work, she and Bruce developed a new level of intimacy in their marriage. Bruce found a full-time job that provided a comfortable income, in response to Tamra's concerns about finances, which ensured that Tamra could take a long maternity leave.

One fall morning, Bruce and Tamra's daughter, Carrie, was born full-term after a long and difficult labor. My work with Tamra didn't end that morning. She decided to continue therapy out of her deep commitment to be a conscious, conscientious and loving parent to Carrie, as well as a partner to Bruce. As a consequence of her ongoing healing work, Tamra also began to improve her relationship with her mother and sister.

Our society usually sweeps the topic of miscarriage under the rug. However, in this chapter, we have seen what potent effect the experience of miscarriage has on your psychological health and, therefore, on future attempts to carry a baby to term. If you have had at least one miscarriage, I urge you to validate your grief by confronting it directly. The miscarriage grief ceremony and following exercise are heartfelt processes for working through your sorrow and self-blame.

SELF-EXPLORATION

HEALING SELF-BLAME ABOUT
MISCARRIAGE THROUGH VISUALIZATION

If you are struggling with harmful self-recriminations about your miscarriage, you may find the following visualization to be helpful:

> Sit in a comfortable position, close your eyes, and allow
> yourself to release whatever tension you may be experienc-

ing in your body. See yourself in your sanctuary. You are surrounded by a bright light that travels across the muscles of your body, releasing any tension still present. The only weight that seems heavy is a large thorn-encrusted sack that the light cannot penetrate. This bag is filled with self-recriminations and blame. Feel the weight of the bag as you walk heavily toward the ocean. Opening the bag, put your hand in and pull out your blaming words and phrases, which you repeat aloud. Then one by one, hurl them—like heavy stones—into the ocean. As the tide carries your hurtful thoughts and blaming words away, you rise and walk away, feeling stronger and lighter in step.

FOR YOUR CONSIDERATION

What feelings were evoked as you read about the women in this chapter who have miscarried? If you have experienced a miscarriage, do you find yourself blocking any hurtful feelings? If so, I encourage you to experience your feelings, including sorrow, anger, and resentment—rather than holding them in your body—by doing the following. Sitting comfortably in your sanctuary, you may want to rub your belly gently and begin by saying, "I feel [supply appropriate word(s)] about my loss." Clients often use words and phrases such as *invalidated, out of control, empty, scared, alone,* and *furious.* You can either verbalize your feelings out loud or write them in your journal, later adding any thoughts and feelings that may occur concerning this experience.

Consider what your mate's feelings were about your miscarriage. How do you feel about the manner in which he responded? Did you share your feelings with him? Did he with you?

NINE

....

Secondary Reproductive Difficulties

The underlying issues affecting women struggling to conceive and hold a pregnancy to term who already have one or more children often are not addressed by health professionals. The woman's doctor will search for physical changes since she was pregnant the last time, but in addition to this necessary examination, I believe it is important that a woman examine the events that have affected her psychologically since she gave birth. If this is your situation, you may wonder why your childhood issues did not prevent your first pregnancy and how they could get in the way now. Consider exploring how your changing life circumstances may be triggering issues that had remained buried during your first pregnancy.

In working with women struggling to have additional children, medical fertility specialists often focus only on physical symptoms that they believe may have manifested or been exacerbated since the birth of the couple's first child. The woman's doctor will research any physical changes in the couple that may be interfering with conception, such as pelvic inflammatory disease, irregular ovulation, or fibroid tumors in the woman, or low sperm count or testicular disorders in the man.[1]

In my experience, I find that it is important for a woman to examine closely the events that have affected her psychologically since she gave birth to truly understand what is happening physiologically to prevent a pregnancy.

Secondary reproductive difficulties generally mean a couple have one or more biological children and yet are unable to conceive again at all or, if they can conceive, to hold another pregnancy to term, after a year of unprotected sex. As you look at your generational family history, negative childhood experiences, and present-day conscious and unconscious conflicts, you may begin to determine what was occurring emotionally at one time that allowed you to have a successful pregnancy, as well as what in your current life may be undermining your fertility. Many of my clients who have been able to identify and resolve their issues have broken through emotional barriers to have additional children; others have come to terms with not having another child, have adopted, or feel satisfied with the child they already have.

An estimated 1.3 million couples struggle with secondary reproductive complications, according to a study by the National Center for Health statistics, and it is likely that there are thousands more.[2] Another government study estimates that of all couples with fertility problems, 60 percent have secondary reproductive problems.[3] Noting the near invisibility of this population, Harnet Simons writes, "It is striking how many couples with secondary infertility report that they don't know anyone else with this problem. The population is less visible than those with primary infertility for two reasons: They are often assumed to be fertile because they have a child, and they are only half as likely to seek medical help as couples who have never had a child."[4]

Of the hundreds of clients in my practice, those who are struggling to have another child are among the most emotionally isolated. Linda P. Salzer, the author of *Surviving Infertility*, writes of this particular loneliness: "It is easy to feel caught between two worlds, fertile and infertile." Salzer believes people tend to be skeptical about whether it is really a serious problem not to be able to have more children. These people, Salzer continues, "cannot understand the tension and sadness that pervade your life when they see that you already have a child. All the disturbing comments made to infertile couples are heard, too, by those with secondary infertility. But in this case, someone may add, 'Well, you've had one baby; you should feel grateful for that.' The comment suggests that the couple has no real reason to be upset."[5]

Among the couples in my practice who are struggling with secondary reproductive problems, about half of them have also experienced primary fertility problems, which makes the situation even more painful for them. "All the horrors of the previous workup and the old tensions within themselves as a couple begin to surface," writes fertility counselor Dianne Clapp. "The pain of the old infertility, largely resolved if the pregnancy resulted in the birth of a child, begins to become acute again."[6] Other couples who had no difficulty conceiving the first time and are now experiencing secondary reproductive struggles are that much more shocked and confounded. One client, Patty, said, "I was under the impression that since I'd had a successful pregnancy the first time, it would be easier the next time. This trouble is causing me anxiety on top of anxiety. Every year, the doctors are saying it's something else. One doctor said that because of my previous history with endometriosis, I'm at high risk for an ectopic pregnancy. I've been so nervous and frightened that I barely have the energy left to take care of my daughter."

Clapp often has found herself in situations where people ask if she has any children, never if she has a child, because people always assume that she has more than one. "The assumptions that are made by society are interesting. One clearly is that if a couple has only one child, it is not because they are infertile, but because they have decided to have only one. In this era of population control such a decision is sometimes sanctioned, but the inference is that it is selfish: you only have one child because you are more interested in your career, or because you really don't enjoy parenting that much....We just do not consider that the couple who has only one child may not do so because of choice."[7]

Perhaps you have grown defensive about wanting to have another child. When introduced to someone who has yet to have a child but dearly wants one, some of my clients have said they feel apologetic for not being "grateful" enough for the child they do have. One young woman told me, "I feel as if I have no right to complain, that I'm being greedy for wanting another child." At the same time, they feel societal pressure to increase the size of their family. Whether it's a car commercial portraying a mother, father, and two children or a restaurant family-sized meal that serves four, the societal message seems to be this: No family is complete with just one child.

As we discussed in previous chapters, feelings of guilt and inadequacy can affect you physiologically and may further compound your existing problems. I have found that many of the women and men in my practice who are struggling to conceive an additional pregnancy feel that their lives are not "safe" enough to have another child. Some women say that their feelings of lack of safety stem from major life changes—whether they be financial, emotional, or physical—that have occurred after their first pregnancy.

Having your first child was in and of itself a major life change with reverberating effects in all areas of your life. Frankly, having a child in today's world is an expensive proposition. Your finances undoubtedly are more strained now than before you had a child, which can leave you feeling financially vulnerable, especially if you were a working woman who left her career to raise her child. Many women feel overburdened with the responsibilities of parenting one child and working outside the home, especially if they feel unsupported by their mates.

One of the major reasons for ambivalence about pregnancy in women struggling with both primary and secondary fertility problems is their fear that they will no longer be self-sufficient. They have worked hard to be economically independent, having lived through the intense frustration of their mothers' economic and emotional dependence on their fathers.

This dilemma was faced by one of my clients, Grace, age forty-five, who teaches law part-time in New Mexico and is married to Louis, a thirty-nine-year-old business executive. They have a six-year-old son, Ronnie, who was conceived before they married. After her son's birth, Grace experienced five first-trimester miscarriages. Although she had undergone extensive testing, including a uterine biopsy and genetic counseling, her reproductive specialist could offer no clear explanation for her difficulty in holding a pregnancy.

During an initial session, Grace was able to pinpoint the differences in her circumstances between when she had a successful pregnancy and her life now that she was experiencing difficulty. "I was not married and I didn't have to worry about how I would be financially supported. I was a successful attorney, had my own home and money in the bank." She became pregnant with Ronnie while Louis and she were on vacation in Hawaii. "I was relaxed and in control of my life then. It wasn't until I was three months pregnant that Louis and I got married. And even during the first half year of my marriage, I still had my own money. But once my maternity leave expired, I didn't want to go back to a sixteen-hour workday. I wanted to be home with my son, and my husband assured me he could handle the major bills if I just worked part-time. But the reality is that I practically have to twist Louis's arm to get two hundred and fifty dollars a week out of him, begging him for every nickel and dime he gives me. I'm always struggling for money, just like my mother did. She had to beg my father for every little crumb. I had vowed I would never give up control over my life. I thought I had made sure I would be different from my mother, but my life is just like hers."

Grace felt her husband was not supportive in her quest for another child. She said angrily, "He only wants to have another baby to please me. He's a wimp." Grace expressed her rage readily, in great contrast to her mother, whom she described as a "sweet, angelic woman who never raises her voice." Her mother had remained serene despite being married for forty years to Grace's father, an emotionally abusive alcoholic who died at seventy-five of lung cancer. Grace's mother, who is fifty-eight, suffers from a chronic respiratory disorder, has high blood pressure, and has recently had a hip replacement. Her "sweet, angelic" posture covered her own unexpressed rage at her life.

Grace's father had three children from an earlier marriage that had ended in divorce. Since he had already fathered three children, he was insistent that Grace's mother devote all her attention to him and not have children. When Grace's mother first became pregnant, he forced her to have an abortion. Grace's mother subsequently had four miscarriages. When Grace was conceived, her mother kept it a secret until her pregnancy was too advanced to be aborted.

Grace was using her husband as a stand-in for her father, which played itself out in her reproductive dilemma. Grace had to break through her fear that men cannot be trusted and that they are abandoners. Healing for her would center around working through her extremely cruel experiences with her father, which would allow for an improved relationship with her husband.

One of Grace's issues with Louis turned out to be a problem with which many of my clients struggle once they have had children: equitable division of household labor. Grace found it hard to get her husband to pitch in with housework and child care. "I work, too, so why should I have to be the housework enforcer?" she asked. For Grace, who had grown up resenting her mother's subservience to a domineering husband, Grace's husband's neglect of household responsibilities made her positively livid.

Sociologist Arlie Hochschild spent years studying the subject of mothers who work outside of the home, and found that even in homes where husbands contribute to the domestic workload, "women worked roughly fifteen hours longer each week than men. Over a year, they worked an extra month of twenty-four-hour days a year. Over a dozen years, it was an extra year of twenty-four-hour days. Most women without children spend much more time than men on housework; with children, they devote more time to both housework and childcare."[8]

Although there are, of course, no more hours in the day than there were before women joined the workforce, working mothers do have twice as much to accomplish. Hochschild found that while women who work outside of the home have higher self-esteem and experience a lower incidence of depression than do homemakers, working mothers get sick more often than their mates and are more likely than any group to be chronically tired and anxious.[9]

Grace began to resolve her issues with her husband, as well as many other areas of conflict in their lives. Six months into our work together, I recommended that she and her husband seek the help of a marriage counselor in their area who could work with them personally.

After she and her husband went into marital counseling, although she did not hold the next two pregnancies, she was able to carry her next pregnancy to term, as they continued resolving their issues, and she gave birth to a second son.

The need to feel emotionally supported and safe is a significant factor in secondary reproductive problems. Some women in conflict-laden marriages have been able to find comfort in church groups and twelve-step programs. For your first pregnancy, you may have found a temporary haven of support that allowed a pregnancy without completely dealing with your emotional childhood issues, but if you didn't resolve them fully, then the blockages will resurface when the support system is gone, and you may feel it is no longer safe to conceive.

One of my clients, Oko, a thirty-seven-year-old social worker at a shelter for battered women in Philadelphia, felt that her anxieties had to do with living in the inner city and feeling frightened when she walked home at night. But she discovered that the root of her fears went deeper.

Oko, a slightly built Japanese-American, described herself as being twenty pounds underweight. She and her husband of five years, Stanley, thirty-two, a contractor, have one child, Sammy, who was three at the time of our first consultation. She had experienced two miscarriages before Sammy's birth and two afterward. Throughout our seven months of working together, Oko grieved over her four miscarriages—utilizing processes described in this book.

Her medical workup also indicated that she had a low progesterone level, which, as discussed earlier, affects a woman's ability to sustain a pregnancy. I knew that Oko's current circumstances were contributing to her hormonal deficiency. We focused our work on what had been occurring in her life during the time when she had experienced a successful pregnancy versus the times when she had had her miscarriages.

Four years before I met her, Oko had participated in a women's group, where she had sought some understanding about her general anxiety and depression. "The first time I was in the group for about ten weeks and then it disbanded. The women seemed very nice, but the leader thought I was very closed and that I didn't fully accept the others. She was right. I didn't feel a part of the group and didn't let the others nurture me." Although Oko conceived while participating in this group, she miscarried in her first trimester. She continued, "Two months later, a new group formed. And this time the experience was different for me because I allowed myself to get closer. I felt the women in this group could give me the support I'd always longed for. And I slowly began to accept their nurturing. I very much wanted to be part of this group, and I was," she explained. Over the course of several months, two other women in the group became pregnant, and so did Oko. This bonding experience gave Oko the safe haven she needed to hold on to her pregnancy. When I asked Oko what the difference was between the two groups, she quickly responded that in the second group, most of the women were older and mothers already.

She remained in the group until the beginning of her third trimester—dropping out when she feared that the highly charged emotional exercises would frighten her child in utero. Eventually, the group disbanded, but it had provided Oko with the long-sought-for nurturing she needed in order to carry her baby to term. During the third trimester of her pregnancy, after she had dropped out of the group, she reported she began experiencing migraines, which are often a flashing road sign that something else is going on.

Migraines cause excruciating pain for an estimated 23 million Americans, 12 percent of the adult population—the majority of them women.[10] These headaches are often attributed to hormonal changes, such as Oko's low progesterone level. But, of course, hormones are strongly affected by our emotional states, and headaches are often the body's response when we bottle up our feelings, particularly anger.

"My doctor told me it was very unusual to have migraines during the third trimester of my pregnancy," Oko said. When I asked her to recall the details surrounding her first migraine, she remembered that she had just mailed her mother a letter to say that she was pregnant. "She lives only a few blocks from me in a home for the mentally ill. I'm the only one of my siblings who has not moved away from our old neighborhood to avoid seeing my mother. I can't let her presence there dictate where I live." Her mother had been in and out of mental hospitals for thirty-two years, and five years earlier, after one of her mother's particularly wounding schizophrenic episodes, Oko had decided to not be in touch with her. "I wrote to her because I was afraid that I would run into her and she would see I was pregnant. I was afraid that if it was a total surprise to her, she'd cause a scene in public. I was afraid she might hurt the baby. She makes terrible scenes." Oko's fear of expressing her rage at her mother for not being "normal" now, when she felt she needed her and while she was growing up, had created the stabbing pain of a migraine.

When Oko was five, her mother was hospitalized for the first time. Her parents' marriage ended in divorce three years later. This double blow—the loss of both mother and father—had long-term consequences for Oko. During her emotional-release work, she consulted her inner guide, who directed her toward a red heart with the word *love* across it. Floating around the heart was a silver safety-deposit box. This vision symbolized Oko's desperate need for love coupled with her need for safety—essentials that had eluded her in childhood.

Blaming herself for the fact that her mother abandoned her, as children do, Oko must have reasoned that if the one person in this world who was supposed to keep her safe was herself so dangerous that she had to be locked away, there could be no safety for Oko if she was anywhere near her mother. That was why she so desperately feared for her baby's safety should she run into her mother in their neighborhood—the same neighborhood she couldn't leave because her mother's pull on her heart remained so powerful. Of course, the sad irony was that with her mother internalized within her, it often must have seemed that she could never feel safe.

Oko's tremendous fears and conflicts concerning her safety as well as that of her son's and the second child that she longed for disrupted her hormonal balance. With her hypothalamus sending danger signals in the form of chemical and neural messages, Oko's body may have responded by not producing sufficient levels of progesterone hormone thus causing an inadequate maturation of the endometrial lining. The embryo then has difficulty implanting and surviving, resulting in a miscarriage.

Oko continued working to release her anger and sadness, utilizing the exercises in chapters 5 and 6. Even though Oko eventually had to discontinue our work due to financial issues, she called me a month later to tell me she was pregnant. Through Oko's visualization, she discovered that the safe place for her and her children was within her.

The emotional toll of secondary reproductive problems hurts everyone in the family, including the existing child. If you are investing a great deal of energy into conceiving again, your child may feel that somehow he or she is not enough for you. If you have a child, consider explaining why you are trying to bring a sister or brother into his or her life. An important component of my work with couples trying to have another child is encouraging them to reassure the existing child of their continued love and devotion, as I did with Sandra, age thirty-five, and her husband, Mark, who is thirty-six.

Before the birth of their daughter, Edith, now six, Sandra had undergone hysteroscopic surgery twice to have benign growths removed from her endometrial lining. Sandra waited for two years before trying to conceive again. Mark had been medically tested and was found to have no fertility problems. While they were trying to conceive again, Sandra's daughter was suffering. "In one month, Edith had the flu and three bouts of ear infections, and just last week the doctor diagnosed her as having an eye infection, which has been recurring. She gets so sick some nights with a quickly escalating fever and then she starts vomiting." It became apparent to Sandra that Edith's medical problems were a reflection of her own ongoing anguish over not only her continual reproductive struggles, but also her mother's tragic death in an automobile accident a year before and her father's marriage two months later. Sandra's anger at her "life of losses" was taking its emotional toll.

If you have a child and are trying to conceive again, be aware of a possible connection between your child's health and your emotional state. If she is getting sick or her behavior changes drastically, these might be signs that your child is reacting to and absorbing your anxiety. As you explore your conflicts and begin to heal, your child will also.

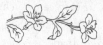

SELF-EXPLORATION

To get in touch with any suppressed emotions concerning your frustrated desires for another child, make a list in your journal of what you are feeling and what you consider to have been insensitive remarks made to you concerning your family status. Also consider what you wish you could say in response. Express your reactions via pillow talk or free-form writing in your journal. It also helps to consider in advance your response to questions such as "Do you have only one child?" You might want to answer nondefensively, "Yes, I do."

FOR YOUR CONSIDERATION

If you have had one or more successful pregnancies and have been unable to get pregnant again, take a moment to consider whether there were some special circumstances that were different for you and your mate prior to, during, and after the birth of your child. Have there been any emotional or life changes since that period of time? Has your sense of security changed? Ask yourself what you need to feel secure and then write your answers down in your journal.

Are you concerned that having another child will threaten your financial independence? How has your financial situation changed over time? What was it like before marriage, after having your first child, and what is it like today?

TEN

Men's Fertility Issues

Although men account for at least half of the people in the United States who are struggling with reproductive problems, they are less likely than women to seek professional help, in my experience. Approximately 20 percent of my clients are men, a third of whom have been medically diagnosed as having sperm-related problems. Very few men seek me out on their own. Most begin working with me because their wives make the initial contact. If you are a woman whose husband could have reproductive problems or might benefit from developing a better understanding of your difficulties as a couple, ask him to read this book, or at least this chapter, which was written with him in mind. Because it is directed to men, from this point on in this chapter, when I refer to "you," I am speaking to male readers.

If you have been hesitant to discuss your feelings with a counselor concerning your part in any reproductive difficulties you and your mate may be experiencing, you should know that you are not alone. Many men often feel uncomfortable in therapeutic situations. A sampling of twenty couples in counseling found that the men had "significantly lower expectations for therapy than the women."[1] Another study determined that men tend to be less verbal than women and harder to reach when therapists utilize traditional approaches.[2] When you consider how children are taught to repress their feelings with dictums such as "Big boys don't cry" and "Don't be a sissy," you can understand why so many men are uncomfortable expressing and releasing their emotions in therapy.

It might encourage you to know that once men move through any initial reluctance to working in my program, they're often quite responsive to the program's nontraditional approaches. A large percentage of my male clients eventually are willing to work through their own frustrations concerning difficulties when their partner has not conceived, and they have achieved major breakthroughs that have positively affected their partner's conception and led to general improvements in their own health. The principles of my mind-body approach to fertility are not untested. Several major health practitioners and medical institutions now recognize that our states of mind and physiological processes are closely linked. The Whole Person Fertility Program[SM] can help you mobilize your inner resources to become your own healer—a particularly important benefit if you have grown weary of having to rely solely on others to help you and your wife conceive.

Even if you are uncomfortable about this nontraditional therapy or have little confidence in therapy, you can still benefit from this process. In fact, many of my male clients have applied the therapeutic principles they learn to all areas of their lives, including work and family. As they release their blocked emotions, all of their creative endeavors prosper, including their procreative capacities. Studies indicate that the instinct to become a parent is not stronger in women than in men or exclusively a female prerogative.[3] Many men in my fertility practice long for babies every bit as much as their wives. Yet just as my female clients benefit from examining conflicts they might have regarding parenthood, the men also are helped. This chapter will help you clarify why you want a child, as well as any fears you may have about changes in your finances and marriage that may be manifesting themselves physiologically.

Frequently, men tell me that their struggles in the medical fertility system—which can be a dehumanizing, demoralizing, and financially exhausting experience—have dampened their desire for fatherhood. In a story detailing the tremendous emotional toll that fertility problems take on a marriage, *Harper's* magazine contributing editor Bob Shacochis wrote of the regimen of hormonal injections he administered to his wife. "Neither of us was brave about the hateful needles, and the tension between us rose; under the stress of hurting her, I'd yell, she'd weep, and for a month the process itself made us adversaries."[4] Shacochis's story called attention to the plight and grief of fertility's often invisible population—men who want to be strong because they believe that is what men should be, when actually they feel vulnerable and powerless. Exhausted and discouraged by the medical system, many of my male clients admit they sometimes feel like giving up on having a baby, although they don't want to disappoint their wives. If this is true for you, try to discuss these feelings with your mate, or with a nonjudgmental friend. Or you might try writing these reflections in a letter to yourself to clarify them. Holding back or denying these feelings can create tension in your body, which can trigger physiological reactions that will undermine your efforts to help your partner conceive and may create distance between you.

Important Factors Affecting Men's Fertility

Until relatively recently, the subject of low sperm counts was considered taboo. In the early fifties, before researchers began examining sperm counts, when a couple was struggling to conceive, the wife was almost always the main focus of the medical inquiry, and she was viewed by everyone from the doctor to the couple as being at fault. "Thirty years ago, if a man produced an erection, along with some sperm, he was presumed to be fertile," according to Dr. Joseph Bellina. "If a couple was childless, neighbors and scientists alike shook their heads and said wasn't that too bad about poor Mrs. Jones. That Mr. Jones needed to make a certain number of sperm to get his wife pregnant was only a vaguely recognized concept."[5]

Today, problematic sperm counts and motility figures—which account for an estimated 60 to 70 percent of male reproductive problems—are still a particularly sensitive issue.[6] One researcher told of sending out questionnaires, with assurances of anonymity, to five hundred men who were thought to have reproductive difficulties. Only fifteen responded. Hoping to learn why so few men were willing to broach the subject, the researcher, Dr. Tracy MacNab, interviewed medical fertility specialists. "The medical clinics explained that their average male infertility patient did not return for a second appointment, often avoiding even the simplest evaluative procedure. A urologist stated that the men whom he dealt with were usually so devastated that they could not talk about what the experience meant to them."[7]

When I asked one of my clients how he felt about being diagnosed as having a low sperm count, he said, "I felt humiliated, like the skinny guy on the beach who has sand kicked in his face." If even a confidential discussion of fertility problems can be so painful, imagine how difficult it might be to have this information become the subject of public discourse. Recently, the actor Tom Cruise threatened to sue the publishers of a German magazine after an article suggested he was "infertile." Cruise's lawsuit sent a clear message. He and millions of other people believe that anything loosely connected to a man's sexual potency, including sperm production, is tied to his image of manliness and power. Throughout the world, people measure manhood according to whether or not men are capable of procreating, protecting, and providing for their families.[8]

One male client insisted his view of himself as a man was not affected by learning that sperm test results indicated that, as he said, "I have ridiculously slow sperm." But when I asked him to explore his reaction to the diagnosis in a drawing, he discovered the depth of his true feelings. Although initially describing his sketches as a joke, he drew a cartoon of Superman, muscles flexed, with a caption beneath it that read: "This is my brother, who has three sons; his sperm moves faster than a speeding bullet." Beneath another sketch, this of a stick figure being hooted at by a group of muscular weight lifters, he wrote, "This is me, sans testicles and zero kids!" He eventually admitted, "This whole business of failing the sperm test makes me feel like I'm not someone whom my wife can rely on. I feel under siege and defenseless." As we continued to work together, he connected his poor self-image to the consistent battering by his "football hero" dad, who had made fun of him for being "bookish." After he dealt with these old emotions and worked to release their hold on his mind-body, his sperm count increased.

Another key issue that comes up for the men in my program is the necessity of becoming a full partner with their wives in their joint attempts to conceive. This includes assuming responsibility in determining your part in fertility difficulties, such as not waiting for your wife to give you information about medical fertility procedures, but asking for or researching them yourself, taking the initiative to become more informed about recommended fertility treatments. You will find that your willingness to be vulnerable and open allows for increased intimacy between you and your mate, which can improve your chances for a natural pregnancy.

Understanding Spermatogenesis

It's always tremendously helpful in mind-body work to develop a full understanding of the interconnection between the emotional and the physical, so that you can realize what it is you need to change in your life. When it comes to spermatogenesis, if you've ever seen a news report featuring an aerial view of the Boston marathon and heard the theme music from the movie *Rocky*, you might begin to imagine what it's like when a quarter of a million sperm "blast into the female genital tract at the rate of 200 inches per second (10 miles an hour)," writes Christopher Vaughan.[9] To reach a woman's fallopian tubes, sperm must travel a distance of nearly three thousand times their length.[10]

To accomplish the rigors of this marathon event, sperm are honed into "lean racing vehicles," complete with tails like "strong whips," with twisting, lashing propeller movements so they can eventually make their way through a woman's vaginal mucus.[11] "As the sperm draw near the egg, they...begin to thrash and flop like fish out of water," continues Vaughan. "This motion may increase the chance that the sperm head will come into contact with the egg's surface. And the egg needs every chance for a sperm to bump into it, because the number of sperm that have made it this far are relatively few. The vast, teeming mass of life that was deposited at the mouth of the cervix has shrunk to a minuscule school of sperm by the time they reach the fallopian tubes."[12]

As the sperm, numbering now fewer than two hundred, float down the fallopian tubes, they undergo a process that allows them to enter an ovum. The cap of the sperm is worn away slowly, releasing enzymes.[13] These enzymes in the few existing sperm that race toward the finish enable them to penetrate two thin layers of cells surrounding the egg. Then the strongest remaining sperm thrusts through the tougher inner layer of the egg—the zona pellucida. When the sperm fertilizes the egg, conception occurs.

To avoid confusion, anxiety, and fear if you are asked to undergo a semen analysis, it is helpful to know what your doctor is looking for. Sperm counts vary greatly in men, according to Carla Harkness. "A sperm count of 20 million or more per cubic centimeter (cc) of semen, however, is usually considered normal (especially in the presence of good motility)." She adds that motility, which is the movement of sperm, is now believed to be "more critical to male fertility than sperm count. A sperm cannot fertilize an egg unless it reaches the Fallopian tube and finds and penetrates the ovum."[14]

Harkness further explains that a standard analysis also includes a "morphology" factor, in which the shape and maturity of a man's sperm is evaluated. "At least 60 percent of the sperm cells should be normal [oval] in shape, contour, and maturity." Irregularly shaped sperm might be doubled-headed, tapered, too small, or too large. The test also includes an evaluation of the amount of sperm ejaculated—one teaspoonful is considered normal—as well as the sperm's liquidity. "If semen remains gelled, poor viscosity is reported."[15] Another test surveys the ability of the sperm to penetrate ovum.[16] Whatever the outcome of your analysis, remember that the mind-body connection is crucial in considering the true meaning of the test results. I do not accept the numbers as the final word about your reproductive health, and neither should you.

The release of the male hormone testosterone, which triggers sperm production, is governed by the hypothalamus-pituitary control center, which is highly sensitive to emotional tension. Studies link heightened anxiety with low sperm counts. Emotional tension can be exacerbated by negative beliefs, behavioral patterns, and conscious and unconscious damaging thoughts, feelings, and attitudes.

Harkness explains that sperm production and release is "coordinated by hormones produced by the testes, hypothalamus, and pituitary gland. The hypothalamus initiates this process by releasing GnRH hormone to the pituitary, which in turn secretes FSH and LH.... Testosterone is produced in response to these hormones, the germ cells within the testes begin to mature and develop tails, and the sperm are released into the epididymis."[17] Once these immature sperm are released, they are nourished for the next two weeks with hormones and fructose so they can maintain motility.

Emotional tension can lower testosterone levels and disrupt sperm production.[18] How much emotional tension does it take to disrupt the process? According to Bellina and Wilson, the mind deals with emotional tension by slowing down the oxygen and blood fed to all but the vital organs such as the heart and brain, and thus the deprived parts of the body begin to suffer. They write, "If we could take sperm counts of men on a battlefield we would probably find them to be extremely low. Modern battlefields can be almost anywhere—behind the corporate desk or in the nuclear power plant, the classroom or on the superhighway, sitting in a courtroom or traveling through outer space."[19] There is a particularly strong connection between men's reproductive abilities and problems and their sense of themselves as professional and economic successes and failures.

Additionally, Dr. Christiane Northrup believes that the seminal fluid a man produces while masturbating in a hospital bathroom before a fertility procedure is of lesser quality because of the emotional tension he may feel.[20] Dr. Lee Spencer, a physician who is also aware of the psychological tension patients undergo during medical fertility diagnosis and treatment, agrees. He says that at least two studies "link psychological stress to decreased or arrested spermatogenesis."[21]

One man, Danny, wrote of his rage at having to "masturbate in a bathroom while looking at the nude, pornographic pictures of a stranger, while my childhood sweetheart, my wife, was in another room praying that I wouldn't let her down again. And I could hear the nurse outside the bathroom. She was waiting to transport my specimen to the laboratory." Danny was taking part in a relatively new medical procedure, called an "intracytoplasmic sperm injection," in which his sperm was injected into his wife's egg. This procedure cost eleven thousand dollars, and reportedly, it has a 24 percent success rate.[22] But Danny said he was so angry about needing medical intervention to get his wife pregnant "that I knew it couldn't work." He was right—it didn't.

Danny and his wife were successful the next time they tried the procedure, after working in the Whole Person Fertility Program[SM], and they now have a son whose birth, Danny says, was "more exciting than receiving an international peace prize." Although Danny's external life had not changed, and although he still had his reservations about the medical procedure, his perception of himself had shifted internally. He had explored his family history to determine which childhood experiences had contributed to his internalized conflicts about becoming a father. The emotional tension he felt in response to his medical procedure had been quite real, but it had also been exacerbated by unconscious reminders of painful events in his life. As he identified the key areas of his life, which were painful and debilitating, he now could feel less like a victim of his experiences with his parents, especially concerning his alcoholic father's very early death.

According to Dr. Nada Stotland, a psychiatrist working with couples involved in the medical fertility system, the standard battery of medical questions, physicals, laboratory tests, and personal inquiries about one's marital life and sexuality leave men feeling emotionally exposed because they are not accustomed to talking frankly about themselves. "The man may develop a feeling of being assaulted, that there has been an invasion of his body, his feelings, his inner self."[23]

The story of Bernard demonstrates the importance of looking closely at childhood experiences that may be exacerbating the level of emotional tension in your body, which then affects your reproductive system. Bernard, age thirty-five, and his wife of fifteen years, Meryl, age thirty-four, are attorneys who practice in Manhattan. During our initial interview, Meryl tearfully spoke of the intense frustration she and Bernard had undergone in trying for thirteen years to conceive. She said, "I cannot give up my dream of having a baby." At the start of our work together, Bernard strongly resisted having his sperm examined. He insisted, "There is nothing wrong with my sperm. If anyone is at fault, it's Meryl." This made Meryl furious, as anyone would be at such a mean-spirited accusation, but also because she had been raised by parents who blamed her constantly for their troubles and often beat her physically.

One partner often blames the other when they have reproductive problems. During the course of our work, however, Bernard realized that he had learned from his mother not to accept responsibility for any problems. As a result of this awareness, he decided to have a medical exam, which revealed he had a low sperm count. This diagnosis left him feeling devastated and fearful of being seen as inadequate. As he intensively worked through these fears, however, he developed a new inner strength. And Bernard and Meryl finally stopped blaming each other.

Many other critical emotional issues affected Bernard and Meryl individually and as a couple. Meryl was intensely fearful of Bernard's anger, but she learned that she had been projecting onto him her fear of her father. When she behaved as a "frightened little girl" or was overly controlling, Bernard grew enraged, saying, "Meryl makes me feel I'm back at home with my mother, who is incredibly manipulative."

Bernard summed up his childhood by saying, "My mother believed that my brother, Mark, could do no wrong and I could do no right." Mark, who is two years Bernard's senior, had also been married for fifteen years and was also childless, more evidence that the childhood experiences of both brothers reflected their parents' negative attitudes toward children, contributing to their childlessness.

As with girls, boys undergo a developmental process of separating and individuating from their mothers—every child's primary attachment figure. Boys and girls both depend on receiving a sense of love and security from their mother, and when the time comes to separate from her, they depend on their fathers to help make that transition to the outside world. "Breaking free from the delicious security of mother love can be a painful rupture for either mother or son," writes Dr. Frank Pittman. "Some boys can't do it."[24] In many cases, mothers are never ready to give up their sons. I have found that when the process of emotionally separating from one's mother is arrested, a man's sperm production can be negatively affected, which is exactly what happened to Bernard. (To better understand the emotional connection between your conscious and unconscious memories and the activities that occur along the hypothalamic route, you may want to read the introduction and look at the "Mind-Body Intercommunication Map" [page 6] if you have not already done so.)

Bernard's mother had a bitter relationship with her husband, who died of a heart attack at thirty-nine, when Bernard and Mark were ten and twelve years old, respectively. That left the brothers with "joint custody" of their mother, serving her emotionally as substitute husbands. She demanded every moment of their time when they weren't in school and tried to monitor every moment of their existence: where they went, with whom, and why. Her rules were exacting. On the few occasions when Bernard arrived a few minutes late to dinner, his mother responded by having an asthma attack, wheezing the words out: "See what you've done to me. I told you not to come home late." While she was impatient and demanding of both brothers, she reserved her most corrosive rage for Bernard.

It was apparent from hearing Bernard's rancorous memories that the effects of being a least-favorite child are enduring. With his mother doling out affection to Mark and cruelly blaming Bernard (who she felt was just like his father), the brothers became locked in an intense rivalry. Bernard was furious about having lost the competition for his mother's love. He once admitted during a session, "I grew up feeling completely undesirable. And I blamed my brother, not my mother, who I now realize actually caused our rivalry."

Mark and Bernard's rivalry continued into their adult life, as their mother refused to relax her hold over them. Even after the brothers married, their mother kept them on twenty-four-hour call, often phoning any time of the day or night to complain about her health or demand that they run errands for her. "Many, many men in this country have grown up in this precarious position; deprived of the love and support of their fathers and forced to rely on their mothers, who, in turn, were relying on them," writes Marvin Allen, a therapist who specializes in men's issues.[25]

Because neither brother wanted to be viewed by their mother as the less responsive son, they acceded to her demands, but at a high price. Bernard's sense that he had given up a part of himself for his mother's love fueled his anger and sense of inadequacy. Their anger united the brothers in an *unspoken* declaration of independence: They refused to make her a grandmother, no matter how much she begged or shamed them.

After Bernard and I had worked together for several months, I asked him again why he felt his unconscious mind might be signaling to his reproductive system that he did not want to conceive a child. He said somewhat defiantly, "I think part of me feels as if it's the one area of my life that I have control over." In truth, as long as he and his brother were locked into their unconscious manifesto against their mother, he really did not have the control over whether or not he would have children. Unhappily, he realized that had he not been reacting to his mother's negative pressure, he would have wanted to have a child. He had spent the last thirteen years fighting against what, as he said, "I want to have."

Bernard was angry at his mother, as well as filled with grief over the loss of his father, but he found it difficult to express any of these emotions. Anyone who has spent years repressing their feelings finds it difficult initially to express themselves in therapeutic or intimate situations. Men, in particular, seldom have had role models for safely expressing their needs. Often separated from a mother's love and nurturance, perhaps deprived of a father's intimacy, and shamed for crying or being fearful in childhood, many young men fashion themselves after what they think men are supposed to be like—devoid of tender feelings and vulnerability, which often is viewed as weak and unmanly. Depending on their personalities, many men are able to express in varying degrees only one real emotion—anger, along with an occasional burst of joy or triumph.

As I continued working with Bernard and Meryl, Bernard remained defensive about any perceived criticism of his parents and redirected the anger he felt for his mother toward Meryl. At first, when he stopped blaming Meryl for his angry outbursts and saw his part in them, he was convinced life would get better if he simply controlled his temper. Then he realized this tactic meant holding his anger in. When he could hold it in no longer, he would blow up at every little incident. Finally, during therapy sessions he agreed to engage in emotional-release exercises, which are included in chapter 5, even though at first he thought the exercises were silly.

For many men, rage is an entry point to the hidden storehouse of their range of emotions. As Marvin Allen explains, many men seem to like this exercise because it allows them privately and safely to direct their pent-up anger at an inanimate object, so no one can get hurt. Striking a cushion with a plastic baseball bat is one way for men to release their anger in a safe manner. Bernard grew adept at venting his anger and sorrow by utilizing this technique. When Bernard was able to release some of his rage, he wept as he expressed his sense of helplessness over his seeming inability to conceive. He gradually was able to experience feelings of grief over the loss of his father as well.

As Bernard and Meryl continued working through their anger and sadness, Meryl found more effective ways to meet her emotional needs, and she changed her responses to Bernard. This was liberating for them both and helped to resolve their long-standing conflicts. In softening his attitude toward his mother, Bernard was able to stop responding to Meryl as if she were his mother. He also became more sympathetic to his mother's real needs for care and responded lovingly to her nighttime calls. This paved the way for major breakthroughs in their lives. Ten months after we had started our work, Meryl and Bernard conceived. Three months later, Bernard reported that his brother and sister-in-law had conceived, as well. Their children are now teenagers.

The Roots of Your Emotional Style

Depending on the quality of a man's relationship with his father, he either emulates his father's emotional style or rejects it. Since your father was an emotional role model for you, it's important for you to explore the range of feelings you saw him express. Would you describe your father, for example, as quietly hostile, cheerful, submissive, exacting and perfectionistic, weak, quiet and withdrawn, scornful, encouraging? Closely consider your father's emotional style. Rebelling against your father's behavior by attempting to act the opposite from the way he did does not mean you have separated yourself from him. You are still tied to your father as a mirror image. It is vital to realize this in order to discover your own feelings. By rejecting your father—the person as well as the role he plays in your life—you also may be rejecting fatherhood.

When I began working with William and his wife, Lee, she described him as being unsupportive and cold during their unsuccessful egg-donor procedure. William described his father as a passive, mild-mannered man who was always making excuses for William's mother, who controlled the family with her seething rage and anxiety attacks. As if he had promised himself he would never be like his father, William grew up with a hair-trigger temper. If Lee voiced her unhappiness or disapproval of a situation, he interpreted it as a personal attack and accused her of being controlling.

William explored the roots of his behavior, and he began to realize how tied he was to his father. He said, "Trying not to be like him is destroying my marriage and obviously interfering with our attempts to have a child. I keep Lee in such an emotional state that her body keeps rejecting the eggs—as if it's not safe for her to bring a child into the world. But the truth is, I don't know any way to stop not being like my father."

He learned that his only way off this proverbial hamster's wheel was to tap into the authentic feelings that lay beneath the cover of the seething rage he had adopted from his mother. But his initial insistence that his anger had nothing to do with his childhood jeopardized his marriage. Yet, in each of their disagreements, he unconsciously converted his wife in his mind to his mother—his primary attachment figure. In turn, Lee saw only William's defensiveness, not the authentic William. Men who view women as their mothers and women who see men as their fathers are common dynamics that keep couples at odds.

During one session, William had a breakthrough when Lee, who works as a pediatric nurse, was describing how she had comforted a little boy who was fearful of his impending surgery. William began to weep. He blurted out, "You give the kids in your hospital more love than me." It was the first time Lee had ever seen William cry, and she was astonished. She embraced him and they comforted each other. Lee said she was shocked to realize that "beneath William's layer of steel, there's someone who hurts as much as I do." Women can get tricked into believing that their mates' stoic, nonemotional stance represents who they really are. That means women seldom get to know or really understand their mates. Realize that if you don't show her your true feelings, the woman in your life may be reacting to your facade.

Fortunately for William and Lee, once William realized the degree to which his emotional reactions were conditioned by his early-childhood memories of his father and as he released some of his repressed anger and sorrow, he learned how to create a warm, supportive environment between Lee and himself. The next time they attempted the egg-donor procedure, it was successful. Now the couple have a thriving baby boy, William Junior.

You can try this for yourself by relating any present relationship conflict back to your childhood experiences, where the original reaction was established. When you are very angry, ask yourself whose voice you really hear being angry with you, or disappointed in you. This can lessen the frequency and intensity of your arguments. As you learn to resolve your conflicts, you can create a more loving, emotional space for pregnancy.

As you have seen, although some of my male clients are uncomfortable experiencing their feelings, that is exactly what you need to do to bring about emotional and reproductive changes. "In order to heal, people can't just talk about their feelings, they have to experience them," writes Marvin Allen. "They can't just complain about their pain and loneliness; they have to cry and grieve and work it out of their systems. In the words of therapist John Gray, 'What you can feel, you can heal.' "[26]

Baby Boomer Men and Their Fathers

Fathers have a profound effect on their sons' lives. "Every boy was supposed to come into the world equipped with a father whose prime function was to be our father and show us how to be men," writes Dr. Pittman. "He can escape us, but we never can escape him. Present or absent, dead or alive, real or imagined, our father is the main man in our masculinity."[27] Boys who grow up inadequately fathered, cautions Dr. Pittman, may never feel comfortable with their masculinity or as fathers.[28]

Almost all of my male clients of the baby boomer generation describe their fathers as weak, cold, rigid, or distant figures, even when their fathers were admired by others for professional or civic accomplishments. Without the necessary parental attachment boys need, they are deeply wounded as men. I know that their fathers knew little about parenting their sons because their own fathers had not been close to them.

In the earliest days of humankind, most of the time fathers spent away from their children was to hunt food for their families. When they were home, they instructed their sons in hunting and other pertinent survival skills. When agrarian lifestyles became the norm, sons toiled beside their fathers in the fields, so that work and family stayed in the same sphere. The Industrial Revolution "was probably the most significant factor in the evolution and decline of the father's role in families," writes Margo Maine, Ph.D. New work requirements kept fathers away from home, leaving mothers with the major responsibility of raising sons and daughters.[29]

During the Great Depression of the 1930s, many of the fathers of the future baby boomers witnessed their own fathers lose their sense of self-esteem and masculinity over not being able to provide for their families. In the period following World War II, however, men who returned from the war entered an American economy that was thriving. Eventually, many of these men would measure their own success as fathers by how much they accomplished financially in the outside world, rather than by the quality of their family life and relationships with their children. During the fifties and sixties, the suburban lifestyle meant longer commutes and shorter periods of parental interaction. All of these changes contributed to millions of baby boomers becoming emotionally disconnected from their fathers' lives. This disconnection was heightened by the rebellion of the sexual revolution and the deferment of marriage and family. Many men saw their fathers give up their dreams, hopes, and desires to become "family" men. One man said, "I made a lot of plans for my life, but the one thing I never planned or wanted before now was a family of my own." Dr. Pittman writes, "The trend is clear; the boys who got fathered want to be fathers, and the boys who didn't get it fear it."[30]

Leo, age thirty-two, a member of a nationally known family of politicians, and his wife, Jennifer, the thirty-one-year-old director of a leading research hospital, had tried for three years to conceive. Given Leo's prolific family, he rather shamefully said, "I have a low sperm count." After questioning his feelings about his diagnosis, I stated that I have never considered that to be the final word. Leo was a bit more heartened by this idea. As I mapped out Leo's family dynamics, I found that Leo's reproductive life was being affected by the aftershocks of his relationship with his father, whose failure in the political arena had been so all-consuming that he had devoted little time to fathering Leo.

Jennifer spoke without hesitancy of the various medical procedures she had undergone, including in vitro fertilization. Leo's doctor believed that his low sperm count was the problem.

Leo and Jennifer had dated since their freshman year at college, during which time Leo had impregnated Jennifer. She said sadly, "I had an abortion. We were just so young then." They both found that, in light of their difficulties in conceiving, they harbored a lot of guilt and shame at having aborted a baby. Leo and Jennifer created a grief ceremony for their aborted child. The grief ceremony allowed them to feel they could begin to move on and make way for another child in their lives. Instructions for creating a grief ceremony of your own can be found in chapter 5.

We examined what had been occurring in Leo's life during his college years that had allowed him to impregnate Jennifer, and what was different now. Leo was actually Leo the third. His father, Leo II, had been named after Leo's grandfather, a political kingmaker. My client's father had been expected to follow in his father's footsteps, but right from the beginning, his father showed him little love and respect, doting on his younger son instead and predicting that one day he would make the family name known worldwide, which is exactly what happened. As for Leo II, "He never had a chance," my client told me. "He said my grandfather was always teasing him about being so much shorter than my uncle or not being as smart or athletic. And my uncle turned against my father, too, never treating him with respect."

Leo's father was an alcoholic, who drank himself to death at forty-five. As soon as his father was buried, the family joined forces and began treating his mother and Leo as personae non grata. Once in college, Leo tried to mend fences with his father's family and reclaim his mantle as heir apparent. "It looked as if they were willing to accept me back into the fold." During the summers, he and Jennifer worked on local campaigns for the family, which was also the time when she became pregnant with their baby, which they aborted. More than a decade later,

Leo was still working for the family, involved in the highest levels in his uncle's campaigns, but his uncle treated him like a glorified office boy.

Leo was affected deeply by the internalized image of his father as a failure. Like his father, Leo had tried to reclaim his family name. But feeling powerless, he instead inherited his father's mantle of "victim." To begin healing, Leo needed to explore his feelings toward his father, his abhorrence of his drunken behavior, the extended family's mistreatment of them both, and his father's early death.

Leo had never expressed his grief over losing his father at such a young age, nor the rage he felt toward his father for dying and leaving him and his mother under the family's jackhammer.

Following several sessions, Leo realized he did not have to live out his father's life, and he began to challenge the family's dictates. He developed a stronger sense of himself and his potency in the world. After eight months of working with the Whole Person Fertility Program^{SM}, Jennifer became pregnant. Leo also made a breakthrough in his professional life. Leo's uncle eventually offered to support him in his candidacy for a statewide office. With his family's support, Leo easily won the election. Leo and Jennifer chose to name their son Benjamin, not Leo. Leo explained, "This will be the first child not to be born buried at least by name under the weight of our family history."

I hope this chapter has helped you understand better your reproductive issues and to consider reading this book in its entirety, if you have not already done so.

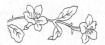

SELF-EXPLORATION

Throughout the book we have discussed how internalized parental voices and critics can determine your attitude about yourself, your attitude toward your body, and your relationship with your spouse. All of these factors affect you reproductively. The exercises in this book are designed to help you and your spouse connect with the aspect of yourself that promotes healing. Besides the following exercises and questions, I especially recommend that you construct your own ephistogram to help you identify intergenerational family patterns and emotional issues that affect you reproductively. You can also engage in emotional-release exercises such as pillow talk and writings, allowing yourself to experience and express feelings of vulnerability and sadness.

As a consciousness-raising exercise, read over the following list of authentic feelings that was compiled by Dr. Charles Whitfield. Consider jotting down the list in a journal or notebook and put a check beside the feelings you have recently experienced.

Under "Joyful Feelings," can you recall experiencing a sense of hope, affection, joy, love, community, relief, involvement, contentment, equality, trust, attraction, curiosity, clarity, support, satisfaction, strength, innocence, pride, contentment, or fulfillment?[31] One man found that although he has won several major awards for his work, he had never felt a sense of pride. Looking back at his father's life, he realized that his father, who was highly regarded in his field, had also been unable to take any pride in his accomplishments. Look at the list again, with an eye for emotions that your father may have expressed that are affecting you negatively today.

On the list of "Painful Feelings," ask yourself if you have recently felt a sense of fear, anger, sadness, hate, loneliness, hurt, boredom, frustration, inferiority, suspicion, repulsion, shyness, confusion, rejection, unfulfillment, weakness, guilt, shame, or emptiness.[32] Again, consider what your father's reactions might be to the same question. If you try any of the emotional-release exercises in this book, review your lists again in a week or so to see if your responses have changed.

I also suggest joining a men's group. You may find that being in the company of men who are working on expressing their feelings and recognizing their own emotional needs will encourage you to do the same.

An exercise that is particularly useful in articulating unspoken feelings or unrealized feelings is letter writing. These letters are not necessarily for sending but as a form of self-expression. For instance, you may try to write a letter as if your father were writing to you, to try to explain the losses he experienced in childhood that affected his fathering. When you have finished, write a letter back to him from you, explaining what you received from him that you appreciate, and also what you did not get from him but wish you had. The more you articulate in your writing, the less you have to carry around inside you.

When you have finished, close your eyes, take a deep breath, and imagine your father putting his arms around you and telling you he loves you and is proud of you. If you feel any resistance to doing this, ask yourself if that is related to never having had (or seldom having had) your father speak to you in this manner or physically embrace you. Allowing yourself to become vulnerable to your emotions and giving yourself the love, affection, and approval you may not have received from either your father or mother is a crucial step in healing. Speak the words of praise you longed to hear from your father. When you have finished, reflect on how this experience felt.

FOR YOUR CONSIDERATION

How did you feel—emotionally and physically—as you read about the issues discussed in this chapter? Consider discussing your fertility problems with a trusted friend or a family member, perhaps one you know who had experienced similar difficulties.

Were you given a label when you were young? Bookish? Jock? Class clown? Nerd? Rebel? How do you feel about being labeled? What about the other men in your family—your father and your brothers? Were you all the same, or did you play different roles? Do you still play that role within your family? What feelings are evoked when you think of the medical tests and procedures that you and your mate have gone through? Can you describe your feelings? Is there an image that comes to mind? Does your description jibe with other situations you've faced in your life? How was your relationship with your parents? Were you a favorite child, or the rebel? How did your mother's treatment of you affect your relationship with your father and with your siblings? Did you imitate your father's behavior style, or did you reject it by rebelling? What would you like to see happen today between your father and your mother? If either one or both are not alive, how do you feel about not being able to change your relationship? Healing past relationships—whether the person is alive or not—is possible and con-siderably helps our own healing process.

PART FOUR

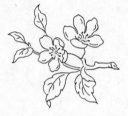

*Healing the
Whole Family*

ELEVEN

Creating Conscious Relationships

Mobilizing anger, rage, hurt, and sadness and learning to release your feelings appropriately is the beginning of an incredible process that ultimately helps set the stage for forgiving your parents and healing all of your personal relationships. The beauty of this work is that it does not prematurely cap these feelings by leading us to forgive those who hurt us before we are ready to do so. Every vestige of hurt and sadness within you will not necessarily be resolved, but by continuing this work, you will move further along the road to true healing and into a place of self-loving.

While reading this book, you have spent much of the time working to identify and understand emotional issues in your life that affect your reproductive health and your life as a whole. You have stirred up many powerful feelings and worked to weaken their hold on you. As you move to a place where you no longer are denying or repressing your anger and resentment, you will be able to embark on a path of feeling compassion for your parents and for yourself because you understand and sympathize with your parents' painful heritage.

Feeling compassion for all the emotional and at times physical suffering we have endured leads to forgiveness that allows you to open yourself to the loving, health-giving aspects of yourself.

By forgiving, however, I am not suggesting that you forget. "There is a word for what happens when we try to forget painful memories instead of dealing with them straightforwardly," write David Stoop and James Masteller. "The word is 'denial.' When we deny what has happened to us, we do not really forget it, in the sense of getting it out of our system entirely. We just pack it up and store it in our emotional deep-freeze....That self-deception never lasts, and it does not free us from the harmful consequences of the past. Though the painful memories are buried, they are still there, still having their effect on us."[1] As we have seen, no one can escape—or is meant to escape—fully the environment and circumstances in which one was raised. We are meant to deal consciously with the challenges our lives present and we're meant to deal consciously with the person we need to forgive—whether it be a parent, a sibling, a mate, or ourselves.

You might be the first person in your family to attempt to break the psychological and emotional chains that are not healthy for any of you. Forgiveness will help you open new ways of communicating, establishing better relationships with your family, mate, and friends. Your courageous act of emotional liberation and forgiveness will also free or restore your ability to conceive consciously, and hopefully consciously parent your child. Forgiveness allows you to make the final step into this healing and receptive place, which is crucial for conception. "Forgiveness helps the one who forgives. When you forgive, the energy that formerly held the resentment in place can be used creatively," writes John Bradshaw.[2] Forgiveness is not a decision, but a process that allows us to see ourselves, our parents, and others as real people.

Perhaps you're thinking, I've already forgiven my father and mother. Many people believe that saying, "I forgive you" makes it true. For genuine forgiveness, however, you first have to have identified the original source of your anger or pain and released some of your suppressed emotions. Only then can you feel compassion for yourself for what you have endured, and, finally, compassion for your parents and family and the hurt they suffered as they were growing up.

Personally, I truly began to understand this when I awoke one morning and sadly realized that my own mother—who had been dead for more than twenty-five years—had to face the terror of her life without the understanding or tools that I had at my disposal. It was an awesome realization and I felt a profound sense of her grief over her painful life for the first time. I had spent so many years of my life in a rage with her. But I now feel more liberated, free to own my right to be who I am—to be womanly, to be at peace, to be a mother, and to write this book. The honesty, clarity, and sense of purpose in my work has grown out of this understanding.

Dealing with Trauma in Your Past

One client whose parents' behavior seemed "unforgivable" was Celia, an incest survivor. Celia's perception of her mother was that she had turned a blind eye to the fact that Celia's father was molesting her when Celia was a child. In fact, for most of Celia's childhood, her mother was hospitalized for a series of nervous breakdowns, brought on by her own unstable childhood. As part of the healing process, Celia had confronted her father, and they eventually had created some sense of peace between them. Even though she was able to forgive the perpetrator, she still could not forgive the act—nor could she forgive her mother for failing to be her protector. As long as Celia was unable to confront her mother, she remained filled with rage.

Eventually, Celia agreed to bring her mother to a session so that the three of us could work together toward a possible reconciliation. Celia recalls, "I was really afraid of going up against my mother because I knew it meant telling her how I really felt. As a child, I had grown accustomed to tiptoeing around her so I would not upset her for fear she would be rehospitalized. My feelings had never come into play— never were allowed to be expressed—never given any notice. Over the years, I'd longed to have a full, healthy relationship with her, but because of her constant need to turn everything around to focus on her, I avoided her. I wanted to protect myself from the hurt, the soulful ache of wanting her undivided attention and never receiving it."

I asked Celia to write up the session—her observations and feelings. She agreed to do so and to have me print her accounting in this book.

It is important to note that when I initially asked her mother what she was feeling being in the session, she responded, "I want a relationship with Celia and at the moment I see a little sliver of light." I was quite moved by her earnestness as well as her courage to face Celia's anger. Her mother, Celia writes, "had six grown children but no grandchildren. I was the first daughter to get married and try to conceive.

"During the session with my mother, I felt like a horrible daughter as I told Mom about the pain I'd held in over the years. I basically told her she'd been a rotten mother! She was shocked and offended, but, at the same time, compassionate and trying to understand me. I told my mother how painful it was to be left at home with my abusive alcoholic father every time she broke down and went into the hospital for a month or more to recoup. No one was there for me. I never got to recoup. I had so much sadness bottled up and pushed down. I was never allowed to feel.

"I finally got the chance to tell my mother about all the pain I felt at not having her there and having to be a little robot when she was around by having to be careful not to upset her so she wouldn't have to go into the hospital again. I told her, through my tears, my worries as a little girl, seeing her depressed and in bed every morning. Just having the repressed words come out of my mouth and freely expressing my feelings was the most liberating experience I'd ever had. I was truly frightened when Mom stood up and declared that she didn't need to hear this and then threatened to leave. Instead of acting like a hopeless, disappointed little girl, I stood my ground and said, 'This is what I expected.'

"Before my mother reached the door, Niravi asked her, 'What would it mean to you to have grandchildren?' I was amazed when [Niravi] said, 'If you stay, the little sliver of light can become a wide open window.' Mom just sat down and her defenses dropped. She cried. I cried. And then for the first time, she was able to connect with me and join forces with me instead of fighting my feelings. It was in one sentence that this revelation was made clear. She said, 'You knew my pain, but I never knew yours.' At that moment, I felt as if my mother finally knew who I was.

"Now that Mom sees and feels what has happened to me, we can end thirty years of silence. The best part of all is that the truthfulness and healing did not end with our mother-daughter sessions. I cannot express in words the wholeness I feel from the steps we took together to heal the past and live a more honest and equilateral life together as mother and daughter.

"Since this breakthrough with my mom, I have felt less desperate in my desire for children. Perhaps the emptiness that usurped the last three years of my life while trying for pregnancy was not the inability to have a child but, rather, my inability to have ever been a child. Although I still want so much to be a mother, my quest for a baby no longer fills my every moment. I have been able to let go of the obsession and have been able to lead a more fertile life."

Celia was fortunate in that she had achieved a personal reconciliation with her mother and was able to remake their relationship into a healthier, more mutually satisfying one. However, you can heal by coming to a place of forgiveness within yourself even if you can't actually reconcile with someone because the person has died or has permanently left your life.

Nicole, a twenty-five-year-old attorney, and I began working together when she was diagnosed with "unexplained infertility" after trying unsuccessfully for two years to conceive with her husband, Michael, a policeman. She said, "I've always been pretty sickly and I've never had lots of energy." I learned that when Nicole was five years old, her father had shot himself in the head and died at twenty-five—the same age Nicole was now. She looked unfazed as she matter-of-factly discussed her father's death. "I forgave him a long time ago. His parents were concentration camp survivors, and the grief they passed on to my father was too much for him to bear."

As we continued to work together, I found that instead of having truly forgiven her father, she was enraged by his suicide but had persistently denied her feelings. When I asked her to write him a letter telling him how angry she was, she responded with a four-page single-spaced letter, detailing just how much she had suffered because of his abandonment. At the same time, while she continued in the Whole Person Fertility Program^{SM}, she explored what her father's life had been like—his unhappy childhood and his miserable shotgun marriage to her mother when she became pregnant.

Several months into our work, Nicole was shocked to discover that before her father killed himself, he had written letters to her and to her brother, which her mother finally acknowledged—although she said she could not find them. This fueled Nicole's long-standing anger at her mother, which she likewise had never expressed. She was obviously angry that her mother never told her about the letters and that she "misplaced" them. Nicole finally expressed her anger, disappointment, and resentment directly to her mother. However, Nicole was thrilled to learn of the letters and said, "I'm so grateful that I was one of the last people on my dad's mind before he died, even when he felt so desperate. He did love me." She began to cry, releasing some of the sorrow that had been within her for two decades. This news of her father's letter was a catalyst that helped her grieving process and she moved toward genuinely forgiving him. With the anger that had such a fierce hold on her psyche loosening, Nicole conceived five months after our initial consultation. She is now six months pregnant. Nicole said, "My dad wasn't a saint or a hero or some evil man; he was simply human."

Creating Conscious Relationships with Your Mate and Immediate Family Members

The quest to forge new and healthier bonds with your parents and siblings is key to creating your own healthy family with your mate and any natural children, adopted children, or stepchildren you may have—a family that provides a welcome, safe, and nurturing environment for all members. As you become aware of the extent to which you repeated your family dynamics with the mate you selected and the love relationship you established, you can more effectively work through your current feelings of anger, hurt, and emotional conflicts, often exacerbated by your joint struggle to conceive. Learning how to express your feelings openly and honestly with each other sets the stage for developing a conscious loving partnership in the process of creating a new life.

Many couples, unfortunately, are unaware of this powerful connection between their parental conditioning and the health of their relationship and so they engage in a silent struggle with each other. The same anger that can undermine your health and emotional well-being can negatively affect your love relationship and undermine your chances for a successful pregnancy.

Given the current increase in stepfamilies, if your mate has children from a previous marriage, pay particular attention to the possibility that this dynamic could present problems for you or trigger earlier memories from your childhood. For example, Ann's husband, Tom, has a sixteen-year-old son, Steven, from a previous marriage. Steven was nine when he moved in with them. Considerable conflict developed between Ann and her stepson, creating intense pressure in her marital relationship with Tom. When she realized she was playing out her painful childhood relationship between her and her two brothers—always having to compete for attention as a child—her reaction to Steven changed, easing the conflict and eventually opening the way for the creation and birth of their baby daughter.

Many of the couples with whom I work need to realize that as they work through family conflicts to consciously conceive, they need to redirect much of the energy they are investing in having a baby toward creating a relationship into which they would want to bring a baby. The Whole Person Fertility Program[SM] as presented in this book can actually offer you both an important opportunity to engage in healing together, even if trying to conceive has strained your love relationship to the limit. In the event that a pregnancy and the birth of your longed-for child does not occur, it will be just as important for the two of you to be able to have created a mutually supportive union, so you can work through (but not deny) your pain.

Two people who have learned the value of a supportive and loving relationship are Annie, a thirty-eight-year-old homemaker, and Larry, age forty-four, a successful entertainment agent. They live just outside of Denver. Annie had experienced four miscarriages before she began working with me. "I've spent the first twenty years of my life struggling with asthma, arthritis, allergies, migraines, and a bleeding ulcer. Doctors have always told me that I would never have children at all," she said. Larry, who has four children from a previous marriage, had been living with Annie for seven years, and she found herself longing for a child.

As an outgrowth of our therapeutic work, Annie began to feel just how much anger she had suppressed all her life—which was endangering her health and well-being. She engaged in emotional-release work and extensive journal writing and learned a healthy and appropriate way to confront her mother, her father, and her husband. As a result, she began to feel healthier, stronger, and personally empowered.

As her relationship with Larry grew stronger, they learned an important lesson above love: Whether we have problems with conception or not, we want to seem strong, competent, giving, and loving, but the fear of being seen as selfish often prevents us from trying to get our needs met within the context of a relationship.

After several long months of trying unsuccessfully to conceive, they continued to devote themselves to improving the level of intimacy between them. Annie said to me at one point, "I've never felt so independent from someone and yet so close to him. Even if we never conceive a child—though I continue hoping we will—I will always be so grateful to you for helping us build the relationship of a lifetime."

A year into the process, Annie conceived and she and Larry decided to marry. Their daughter, Clarice, has enhanced their union. Annie said recently, "When I wake up in the morning to Clarice's delicious smile and next to a true partner I never thought I'd have, I remind myself that we can have it all. That's my new family motto: Everything is possible when two people who love each other work together."

I asked both Annie and Larry to write letters to you, the reader, so you can hear in their own words the tremendous importance of creating a loving and supportive relationship, especially when you are trying to conceive.

Annie's Letter: "Wanting a Baby Was My Initial Inspiration"

Through my work in psychotherapy, I discovered I carried the self-image of the sick and weak child within me. I was living it out, and projecting it onto myself as powerfully as it had been taught me at age four. I also discovered I was projecting my parents' point of view of me—critical, childish, helpless, stupid—onto Larry. And I was acting with him as I was taught to be in a relationship—the silent, suffering, but always sunny playmate and martyr. It was suffocating me and alienating him. Plus, I was scared to death of him! I would alter my wants, needs, and all forms of self-expression to make him comfortable. It sounds ridiculous to be a grown woman so afraid of anyone around me being angry that I would change my behavior, my joy as well as my pain, to keep him from leaving me. I was re-creating my childhood every day.

I had always considered myself an easygoing, high-functioning, and joyful person who carried little tension in my body, like my dad. Through the Whole Person Fertility Program^{SM}, I saw I was a twenty-four-hour-a-day pressure cooker of unconscious, old, and unexpressed feelings. My so-called easygoing dad had diabetes, high blood pressure, heart disease, and kidney disease before he died of cancer at seventy-three. He had been my role model on many levels, and I realized I had a lot of hard work to do to heal my body and my life.

Wanting a baby was my initial inspiration. Then I

began to see how the family patterns I was carrying were squashing me and tearing up my relationship, and I decided to put my energies on improving our lives together. It was a painful road home, reexperiencing the wounds of my childhood and things I had been taught about myself—weak, barren, selfish, undeserving, ugly—the list is long. As a child, in my relationship with my dad, I was the one who was charged with being his emotional caretaker. I put a lot of my own needs, wants, and desires second to what my father wanted, and I projected that same relationship onto Larry. I realized that my tension was not about whether I agreed to all of my husband's requests. It was about getting in touch with what I needed and being able to express myself openly. I needed to be able to say out loud, "I need this right now." To have someone respect my needs is a very new experience for me.

The whole idea was that there wasn't necessarily something wrong with just my reproductive tract, as is so often thought when we go to a physician and try to deal with fertility problems. It had something to do with my whole way of being in the world and my relationship to myself and to Larry. There were emotional issues blocking my ability to carry a child to term.

Today I don't experience the gut-wrenching level of fear and panic that I used to, even in scary or challenging situations. I am no longer living at an unconscious level, the servant-healer with no needs of her own.

Larry's Letter: "We Had Been in a Dance I Wasn't Even Conscious Of"

I feel that what held Annie back from expressing her feelings earlier in our lives was the fear that I would abandon or reject her, or that I wouldn't meet her needs. I feel she was projecting that onto me. I didn't have any plans to run *away. As we continued working with Niravi, our life together grew so strong, I knew I was in this for the long run. I came to see that we had been in a dance I wasn't even conscious of. Also, having experienced continual loss through the miscarriages was really very stressful, and I know for myself that I struggled with blame. I felt a helplessness and powerlessness that was quite painful.*

Early on, when I began working with Niravi, I felt extremely threatened. She constantly challenged me to express my authentic emotions. This has always been shaky ground for me. My dad's opinion of therapy was that too much introspection caused trouble, and so I, too, shared this opinion.

Then suddenly, here was my sweet angel Annie in therapy, expressing emotions I wasn't sure I wanted to hear. I started to see that things between us were really going to change, and God only knew what she was going to unearth in herself! I was afraid that Annie would turn into somebody I didn't know. And I think that most people are afraid of therapy on that level. But when I, too, began working with Niravi, she helped me to understand that the quality of our relationship could actually influence whether or not Annie could carry our child to term.

Our desire for a child and my love and trust of Annie and her intuition meant I became willing to turn over every stone to find out what was in the way emotionally. That took me into the fire of the Whole Person Fertility Program^{SM}'s mind-body process. As I did the work, I found it to be the deepest, most challenging form of therapy I've ever known. Today, I am so thankful for our daughter, Clarice, and the kind of loving, supportive marriage I never thought possible.

Throughout this book, we have explored how unconscious, destructive family patterns not only have been blocking your ability to conceive but also have been affecting all of your relationships as you have responded to life through reflexive inherited behaviors. With the work you have done uncovering and purging these negative influences, you will be able to build more authentic relationships with the people who are important to you—your parents, other family members, and your mate—and to become a conscious parent to the child you hope to have (and perhaps have now).

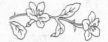

SELF-EXPLORATION

INTERNALIZING A HEALTHY MOTHER AND FATHER

Learning to consciously reparent yourself as you seek to conceive consciously is truly embarking on a healing journey. In your willingness to become aware of the issues that might be blocking your conception, you have had to come face-to-face with many painful childhood experiences and the negative parental conditioning that you have internalized, affecting your life today.

Perhaps you feel that you never will receive the parental love your emotional child within needs and wants. This exercise provides an important and unique opportunity for you to begin to lovingly reparent yourself by combining within yourself the best traits of your parents as they really were with the nurturing traits that you needed but that they were unable to provide.

Begin this exercise by describing in your journal the traits that you most admire in your mother. The list can be as long as you want. Then list your father's best traits. At the bottom of the two lists, add in characteristics that you *wish* they had demonstrated and that you want to develop within yourself.

When you have finished, locate two small objects to represent each of your parents, such as photos, a piece of jewelry, a figurine, a scarf, a bottle of perfume or shaving lotion, a kitchen utensil—whatever you pleasurably associate with each parent. The objects are meant to serve as representations of the maternal and parental aspects of yourself. Place your mother object a few feet away to your left and your father object a few feet to your right, so that if you were seated and stretched your arms to your right and left, you could touch the objects with your fingertips. Visualize imaginary lines running between the objects and yourself as they form a triangle.

Sit comfortably, close your eyes, and take several deep breaths as you enter your inner sanctuary and connect with your inner guide (see chapter 5). Feel the warmth radiating from your guide as your tension melts away. As you talk with your inner guide, explain that you would like to develop (name each trait) of your internalized mother and father. See your guide pointing to two figures in the distance. As you begin walking toward them, you see it is your mother and father standing at the entrance of a cave, cabin, cottage, or any dwelling that feels right for you.

As you approach, they move closer to you. Your parents shine with good health and vibrancy. See their happiness and excitement as they watch you approach. As they welcome you with warm embraces, allow yourself to recall memories of your most wonderful moments with them. Your mother shares with you a beautiful painting she has just completed of your inner sanctuary. She has used her mother's intuition to know and understand every detail of the environment you require to feel joyful and at peace. As you grasp her hand, feel her tremendous strength, love, and intelligence shining in her eyes.

Observing your father, see him as protective, strong, and demonstrative. When there has been trouble in the past, his skills as a master strategist have ensured your survival. He will serve as a strong bridge for you to climb to the outside. By the warmth of the fire you have built in your sanctuary you share with your parents the best of who you are and your dreams of all that you want to be. Tell them of your longing to conceive a baby that you consciously want to parent. They listen attentively. Hear their voices as they tell you of their love, admiration, and pride in you.

See yourself joining hands with your internalized parents—each standing equidistant from you. Feel the balance and harmony of this triangle: separate but unified, no one point in the middle, no one point alone.

See yourself leaving your sanctuary with your inner guide, who is pointing to a mountain in the distance. Hear your inner guide explain that she or he will remain by your side as you climb the mountain, and that to prevail, you will utilize the skills and attributes that are the highest aspects of your internalized mother and father. Moving across a field, the warmth of your parents within you, feel yourself opening to the creative forces of the universe. Move up the mountain, feeling exhilarated. Breathe deeply. Notice how you are climbing. Is it with ease? Laborious? Take some deep breaths. As you descend the mountain, nearing the bottom, see yourself slowly opening your eyes and feeling the strength of your whole self.

On days when you feel the need for this exercise, just close your eyes and visualize this scene. In truly being able to honor the mother and father who are within you, your "internalized war" eases, creating more peaceful and receptive space for you to live in mind-body unity.

Epilogue: No Endings, Only Beginnings

As you continue on your journey, you may begin to wonder, How will I know when to stop trying to conceive and birth a healthy baby? There is no easy answer to this question. I do know the truth lies within you. Sitting quietly with your mate and asking for inner guidance will be very helpful in making your decision. When your mind and body and heart are speaking the same language, you will know just how long to continue in your efforts to conceive.

Many women and men in my practice have conceived, and some have not. But through this important work, they have all come to a place of healing so that they are more open to experience the richness of life. The highest goal of my process is for you to reach a place of self-love, self-acceptance, and self-nurturance that allows for inner peace. My greatest hope is that this book has moved you further along the path to the profound healing inherent in the Whole Person Fertility Program^{SM}.

When hearing that my coauthor and I had finished our manuscript, one of my clients asked what I'd like to see happen with this book. I didn't have to think long to answer. Over the last five years, as I have assembled considerable research in preparation for writing the book, I have envisioned an international network of mind-body fertility therapists, people who have been trained in the concepts of the "whole person" approach to reproductive health. It is to this end that I intend to concentrate my energies in the forthcoming period. I also hold a vision that members of the medical system will move their sights higher, and that no medical fertility practice will be considered complete without a therapeutic support staff that would treat each patient as the unique individual that she or he is. This would mean that when searching for the reasons a person is not conceiving, doctors would work in conjunction with trained therapists who are helping each patient explore how his or her generational history could be affecting any reproductive difficulties the person is experiencing. Finally, I hope that every person, whether or not she conceives and gives birth to a baby, will complete the search with a sense of wholeness, peace, and hopefulness about the present and future.

I trust that the concepts and ideas generated by the stories and supporting data in this book will help create a growing awareness and understanding of the interrelatedness of the mind, emotions, body, and our spiritual selves. In healing our intimate relationships, we can open ourselves to trusting the innate wisdom of our bodies as we reclaim our natural ability to procreate. In challenging the myths of the separation of the mind and body, I hope more women will be able to make a reasoned assessment of their reproductive issues and options without succumbing to the fears being generated today about "time running out."

As you have observed throughout this book, there is time in life for all your dreams. As I near the completion of my five-year vision to write this book, I realize how much of my own life has changed as I have gained the self-love and self-assurance I'd always worked and hoped for.

At one point in my life, my ultimate goal was to make this a better world for my children. Then I wanted to improve it for my grandchildren. Now I am working to improve the world for my great-grandchildren. May they, as well as you, know the joy of living consciously, conceiving consciously, and parenting consciously.

Endnotes

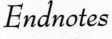

PROLOGUE

1. Elaine Appleton, "Woman to Woman With Dr. Christiane Northrup," *Body Mind Spirit*, November/December, 1994, p. 29.

INTRODUCTION: THE MIND-BODY CONNECTION IN REPRODUCTION

1. Barbara Hoberman Levine, *Your Body Believes Every Word You Say* (Lower Lake, California: Aslan Publishing, 1991), p. 37.

2. Lewis E. Mehl, M.D., Ph.D., *Mind and Matter: A Healing Approach to Chronic Illness* (Berkeley, California: Mind/Body Press, 1986), p. 154.

3. Christiane Northrup, M.D., *Women's Bodies, Women's Wisdom: Creating Physical and Emotional Health and Healing* (New York: Bantam Books, 1994), p. 3.

4. Frank Minirth, *The Power of Memories: How to Use Them to Improve Your Health and Well-Being* (Nashville, Tennessee: Thomas Nelson Publishers, 1995), p. 37.

5. Daniel Goleman, "Ability to Recall Events Tied to Fight-or-Flight Reaction," *San Diego Union-Tribune*, October 26, 1994.

6. Daniel Goleman, *Emotional Intelligence* (New York: Bantam Books, 1995), p. 60.

7. Ibid.

8. Ibid., p. 61.

9. Ibid., p. 10.

10. Information contained under the section "The Science of Emotion, Memory, and Physiological Responses" was compiled under the direction of Dr. Ann Maugeri.

11. David R. Rubinow and Catherine A. Roca, "Infertility and Depression," *Psychosomatic Medicine* 57 (1995): 515.

ONE. WHY SO MANY BABY BOOMERS ARE EXPERIENCING FERTILITY PROBLEMS

1. Sylvia Ann Hewlett, *The Aberrant 50s, A Lesser Life: The Myth of Women's Liberation in America* (New York: William Morrow, 1986), p. 236.

2. Ibid.

3. Ibid., p. 232.

4. Ibid., p. 249.

5. Ann Taylor Fleming, *Motherhood Deferred* (New York: Ballantine Books, 1994), p. 32.

6. Bernard Asbell, *The Pill: A Biography of the Drug That Changed the World* (New York: Random House, 1995), p. 7.

7. Fleming, p. 90.

8. Gail Sheehy, *New Passages: Mapping Your Life Across Time* (New York: Random House, 1995), p. 36.

9. Philip Elmer-Dewitt, "Now for the Truth About Americans and Sex," *Time*, October 17, 1994, p. 68.

10. Lynn Rosellini, "Sexual Desire," *U.S. News & World Report*, July 6, 1992, p. 62.

11. Asbell, p. 28.

12. Ibid., p. 44.

13. Ibid., p. 169.

14. Dewitt, Philip Elmer, "Now for the Truth About Americans and Sex," *Time*, October 17, 1994, p. 70.

15. Dr. Robert R. Franklin and Dorothy Brockman, *In Pursuit of Fertility* (New York: Henry Holt, 1990), p. 265.

16. Sheehy, *New Passages*, p. 15.

17. Virginia Rutter, "Who Stole Fertility?" *Psychology Today*, March/April 1996, p. 48.

18. Patricia McBroom, *The Third Sex: The New Professional Woman* (New York: Paragon House, 1992), p. 258.

19. Ibid., p. 27.

20. Ibid., p. 29.

21. Hewlett, *The Aberrant 50s*, pp. 249–250.

22. Clarissa Pinkola Estés, Ph.D., *Women Who Run with the Wolves: Myths and Stories of the Wild Woman Archetype* (New York: Ballantine Books, 1992), p. 115.

23. Christiane Northrup, M.D., *Women's Bodies, Women's Wisdom: Creating Physical and Emotional Health and Healing* (New York: Bantam Books, 1994), p. 352.

24. Linda Schierse Leonard, *The Wounded Woman* (Boston: Shambhala, 1982), p. 17.

25. Monique Burns, "A Sexual Time Bomb: The Declining Fertility Rate of the Black Middle Class," *Ebony*, May 1995, p. 74.

26. Brenda Lane Richardson, "The Dilemma of the Black Middle Class," *APF Reporter*, Summer 1986, p. 7.

27. Burns, "A Sexual Time Bomb," p. 75.

28. Ibid.

29. Ibid., p. 196.

30. Northrup, *Women's Bodies, Women's Wisdom*, p. 169.

31. Ellis Cose, *The Rage of a Privileged Class* (New York: HarperCollins, 1993), p. 38.

32. April Martin, *Lesbian & Gay Parenting Handbook* (New York: HarperCollins, 1993), p. 3.

33. Ibid., p. 6.

34. Abraham H. Maslow, *Motivation and Personality* (New York: Harper and Row, 1970), p. 43.

35. June Gould, *The Writer in All of Us: Improving Your Writing Through Childhood Memories* (New York: Penguin, 1991), p. 2.

TWO. WHO SAYS I AM TOO OLD?

1. Christiane Northrup, M.D., *Health Wisdom for Women*, vol. 2, no. 7 (July 1995), p. 4.

2. Christiane Northrup, M.D., *Women's Bodies, Women's Wisdom: Creating Physical and Emotional Health and Healing* (New York: Bantam Books, 1994), p. 379.

3. Gail Sheehy, *New Passages: Mapping Your Life Across Time* (New York: Random House, 1995), p. 61.

4. Northrup, *Women's Bodies, Women's Wisdom*, p. 441.

5. F. Gary Cunningham, M.D., and Kenneth J. Leveno, M.D., "Childbearing Among Older Women," *The New England Journal of Medicine*, October 12, 1995, p. 1002.

6. Beth Weinhouse, "Is There a Right Time to Have a Baby?" *Glamour*, May 1994, p. 285.

7. Ibid.

8. Ibid., p. 251.

9. Elizabeth Davis, "Birth Over 40," *Mothering*, Spring 1994, p. 78.

10. Virginia Rutter, "Who Stole Fertility?" *Psychology Today*, March/April 1996, p. 49.

11. Leslie Laurence, "Pregnancy After Forty," *Town & Country*, August 1995, p. 86.

12. Northrup, *Health Wisdom for Women*, p. 4.

13. Laurence, "Pregnancy After Forty," p. 88.

14. Carla Harkness, *The Infertility Book: A Comprehensive Medical and Emotional Guide* (Berkeley, California: Celestial Arts, 1992), p. 105.

15. Northrup, *Health Wisdom for Women*, p. 4.

16. Ibid.

17. Sharon Begley, "The Baby Myth," *Newsweek*, September 4, 1995, p. 40.

18. Rutter, "Who Stole Fertility?" p. 49.

19. Barbara Baker, "'Older' Women Make the Grade as Oocyte Donors," *ObGyn News*, July 15, 1994, p. 24.

20. Harkness, *The Infertility Book*, p. 189.

21. Ibid.

22. Ibid., p. 216.

23. Sheehy, *New Passages*, p. 191.

24. Deepak Chopra, M.D., *Ageless Body, Timeless Mind: The Quantum Alternative to Growing Old* (New York: Harmony Books, 1993), pp. 5, 7.

THREE. MAKING THE CONNECTION BETWEEN YOUR EMOTIONS AND FAMILY AND YOUR FERTILITY

1. Leo Madow, M.D., *Anger* (New York: Macmillan Publishing, 1972), p. 71.

2. Jane E. Brody, "Emotions Found to Influence Nearly Every Human Ailment," *New York Times*, May 24, 1983, p. C8.

3. Harriet Lerner, *The Dance of Anger* (New York: Harper and Row, 1985), p. 96.

4. Ibid., p. 5.

5. Elliott Dacher, M.D., *PNI: The Mind/Body Healing Program* (New York: Paragon House, 1991), p. 20.

6. Bob Hoffman, *No One Is to Blame: Freedom from Compulsive Self-Defeating Behavior* (Oakland, California: Recycling Books, 1988), p. 19.

7. Joan Borysenko, "The Therapy That Changed My Life," *Changes*, April 1994, p. 43.

8. Clarissa Pinkola Estés, Ph.D., *Women Who Run with the Wolves: Myths and Stories of the Wild Woman Archetype* (New York: Ballantine Books, 1992), p. 180.

9. Researchers Judith Dunn, Robert Plomin, and Margaret Nettles discussed sibling development in "Consistency of Mothers' Behavior Toward Infant Siblings," *Annual Progress in Child Psychiatry and Development*, 1986, p. 25.

10. Hoffman, *No One Is to Blame*, p. 34.

11. Barbara Mathias, *Between Sisters* (New York: Dell Publishing, 1992), p. 43.

12. Ibid., p. x.

13. Ibid., p. ix.

14.   Dr. Kevin Leman, *The Birth Order Book* (New York: Dell Publishing, 1985), p. 45.

15.   Ibid., p. 103.

16.   Ibid., pp. 58–59.

17.   Ibid., p. 58.

18.   Lerner, *The Dance of Anger*, p. 118.

FOUR. THE WHOLE PERSON FERTILITY PROGRAM[SM] IN ACTION

1.   Alexandra's diagnostic tests included an endometrial biopsy—a small part of her endometrium was examined under a microscope; a postcoital test—her cervical mucus was examined shortly after intercourse to determine the survival of sperm inside her body; a hysterosalpingogram—dye was injected into her uterus to aid in examining the uterus and fallopian tubes; a laparoscopy—a minuscule telescope was inserted through her navel into her pelvic cavity. In an intrauterine insemination, her husband's sperm were washed and inserted directly into her uterine cavity. Pergonal is an ovulation drug.

2.   Emma Segal, "Infertility: Is He the Cause?" *New Woman*, March 1996, p. 68.

3.   Serge King, *Imagineering for Health: Self-Healing Through the Use of the Mind* (Wheaton, Illinois: Theosophical Publishing House, 1981), p. 84.

4.   Thomas Verny, M.D., with John Kelly, *The Secret Life of the Unborn Child* (New York: Bantam, Doubleday, Dell, 1981), p. 13.

5.   Ibid., p. 29.

6.   Ibid., p. 13.

FIVE. THE HEALING JOURNEY

1.   Dr. Dean Ornish, *Dr. Dean Ornish's Program for Reversing Heart Disease* (New York: Ballantine Books, 1990), p. 82.

2.   Ralph Blum, *The Book of Rune Cards* (New York: St. Martin's Press, 1989), p. 176.

SIX. COMMUNICATING WITH YOUR MIND-BODY

1.   John J. Stangel, *The New Fertility and Conception: The Essential Guide for Childless Couples* (New York: New American Library, 1988), p. 149.

2.   John Bradshaw, *Family Secrets: What You Don't Know Can Hurt You* (New York: Bantam Books, 1995), p. xiii.

3.   N. Caccia, J. M. Johnson, G. E. Robinson, and T. Burna, "Impact of Prenatal Testing on Maternal-Fetal Bonding," *American Journal of Obstetrics and Gynecology*, October 1991, p. 1122.

SEVEN. MENSTRUAL AND OVULATION IRREGULARITIES

1. Christiane Northrup, M.D., *Women's Bodies, Women's Wisdom: Creating Physical and Emotional Health and Healing* (New York: Bantam Books, 1994), p. 97.

2. The details in this section were compiled from the following sources: Jonathan Miller and David Pelham, *The Facts of Life* (New York: Viking Penguin, 1984); Carla Harkness, *The Infertility Book: A Comprehensive Medical and Emotional Guide* (Berkeley, California: Celestial Arts, 1992), pp. 105–107; and Northrup, *Women's Bodies, Women's Wisdom*, pp. 196–197.

3. Harkness, *The Infertility Book*, p. 106.

4. Ibid., p. 129.

EIGHT. MISCARRIAGES: "HOW CAN I HOLD MY PREGNANCY TO TERM?"

1. Dinora Pines, "Pregnancy, Miscarriage and Abortion, A Psychoanalytic Perspective," *International Journal of Psychoanalysis* 71 (1990): 302.

2. Christiane Northrup, M.D., *Women's Bodies, Women's Wisdom: Creating Physical and Emotional Health and Healing* (New York: Bantam Books, 1994), p. 363.

3. Laura Mosedale, "Miscarriage: The Silent Loss," *Child*, June/July 1993, p. 85.

4. Jonathan Scher and Carol Dix, *Preventing Miscarriage: The Good News* (New York: HarperCollins Publishers, Inc., 1991), p. 8.

5. Robert J. Weil, M.D., and C. Tupper, as quoted in Northrup, *Women's Bodies, Women's Wisdom*, p. 362.

6. Grolier Electronic Women's Encyclopedia, Grolier Electronic Publishing in conjunction with Aaron Freedman, M.D. (Danbury, Connecticut, 1995).

7. Niels H. Lauersen, M.D., Ph.D., and Colette Bouchez, *Getting Pregnant* (New York: Ballantine Books, 1992), p. 214.

8. Sharon Begley, "The Baby Myth," *Newsweek*, September 4, 1995, p. 43.

9. Ibid.

10. Northrup, *Women's Bodies, Women's Wisdom*, p. 30.

11. Lauersen and Bouchez, *Getting Pregnant*, p. 214.

12. Mosedale, "Miscarriage: The Silent Loss," p. 90.

13. Ernest Rossi, *The Psychobiology of Mind-Body Healing* (New York: W.W. Norton, 1986), p. 144.

14. Mosedale, "Miscarriage: The Silent Loss," p. 88.

15. Jack M. Stack, "The Psychodynamics of Spontaneous Abortion," *American Journal of the Orthopsychiatric Association*, January 1984, p. 162.

16. Scher and Dix, *Preventing Miscarriage*, p. 12.

17. Charles Whitfield, M.D., *Healing the Child Within* (Deerfield Beach, Florida: Health Communications, Inc. 1987), p. 86.

18. Ibid., p. 87.

19.   Stack, "The Psychodynamics of Spontaneous Abortion," p. 163.

20.   Phyllis C. Leppert and Barbara Pahlka, "Grieving Characteristics After Sponta-
      neous Abortion," *Obstetrics and Gynecology*, July 1984, p. 119.

21.   N. Caccia, J. M. Johnson, G. E. Robinson, and T. Burna, "Impact of Prenatal
      Testing on Maternal-Fetal Bonding," *American Journal of Obstetrics and Gyne-
      cology*, October 1991, p. 1124.

22.   B. Stray-Pedersen and S. Stray-Pedersen, "Recurrent Abortion: The Role of
      Psychotherapy" in Bear, R. W., and F. Sharp, eds., *Early Pregnancy Loss—Mech-
      anisms and Treatment* (London, England: The Research Press, 1988), pp.
      433–40.

NINE. SECONDARY REPRODUCTIVE DIFFICULTIES

1.   Sheldon H. Cherry, "Secondary Infertility," *Parents' Magazine*, May 1992,
      p. 205.

2.   Felicia E. Halpert, "When You Can't Conceive Again," *Parents' Magazine*, Sep-
      tember 1994, p. 29.

3.   Linda P. Salzer, *Surviving Infertility* (New York: HarperCollins, 1991), p. 218.

4.   Harriet Fishman Simons, *Wanting Another Child: Coping with Secondary Infer-
      tility* (New York: Simon & Schuster, 1995), p. 3.

5.   Salzer, *Surviving Infertility*, p. 219.

6.   Dianne Clapp, "Secondary Infertility," *Technology and Infertility: Clinical, Psy-
      chosocial, Legal, and Ethical Aspects*, ed. Michelle M. Seibel (New York:
      Springer-Verlag, 1992), p. 313.

7.   Ibid.

8.   Arlie Hochschild, with Anne Machung, *The Second Shift* (New York: Avon
      Books, 1989), pp. 3–4.

9.   Ibid., p. 4.

10.   Patricia Bosworth, "Can the Mind Really Heal the Body?" *Self*, February 1996,
      p. 126.

TEN. MEN'S FERTILITY ISSUES

1.   Marvin Allen and Jo Robinson, *Angry Men, Passive Men* (New York: Fawcett
      Columbine, 1993), p. 128.

2.   Ibid.

3.   Margo Maine, *Father Hunger* (Carlsburg, California: Gurze Books, 1991), p. 39.

4.   Bob Shacochis, "Missing Children," *Harper's*, October 1996, p. 61.

5.   Joseph H. Bellina and Josleen Wilson, *You Can Have a Baby* (New York: Crown
      Publishers, 1985), p. 79.

6.   Carla Harkness, *The Infertility Book: A Comprehensive Medical and Emotional
      Guide* (Berkeley, California: Celestial Arts, 1992), p. 244.

7. Samuel Osherson, *Finding Our Fathers* (New York: Ballantine Books, 1986), p. 115.

8. Frank Pittman, *Man Enough* (New York: Berkeley Publishing, 1993), p. xiv.

9. Christopher Vaughan, *How Life Begins* (New York: Random House, 1966), p. 28.

10. Harkness, *The Infertility Book*, p. 110.

11. Vaughan, *How Life Begins*, p. 28.

12. Ibid., p. 30.

13. Harkness, *The Infertility Book*, p. 111.

14. Ibid., p. 240.

15. Ibid., pp. 240–241.

16. Ibid., p. 242.

17. Ibid., p. 110.

18. Niels H. Lauersen, M.D., Ph.D., and Colette Bouchez, *Getting Pregnant* (New York: Ballantine Books, 1992), p. 48.

19. Bellina and Wilson, *You Can Have a Baby*, p. 87.

20. Christiane Northrup, M.D., *Women's Bodies, Women's Wisdom: Creating Physical and Emotional Health and Healing* (New York: Bantam Books, 1994), p. 359.

21. Lee Spencer, "Male Infertility: Psychological Correlates," *Post Graduate Medicine*, February 1, 1987, p. 223.

22. Denise Grady, "How to Coax New Life," *Time*, Fall 1996, p. 38.

23. Nada L. Stotland, ed., *Psychiatric Aspects of Reproductive Technology* (Washington, D.C.: American Psychiatric Press, 1990), p. 27.

24. Pittman, *Man Enough*, p. 153.

25. Allen and Robinson, *Angry Men, Passive Men*, p. 78.

26. Ibid., p. 130.

27. Pittman, *Man Enough*, p. 107.

28. Ibid., p. 113.

29. Maine, *Father Hunger*, p. 29.

30. Pittman, *Man Enough*, p. 275.

31. Charles Whitfield, *Healing the Child Within* (Deerfield Beach, Florida: Health Communications, Inc., 1989), p. 84.

32. Ibid.

ELEVEN. CREATING CONSCIOUS RELATIONSHIPS

1. David Stoop, M.D., and James Masteller, M.D., *Forgiving Our Parents, Forgiving Ourselves* (Ann Arbor, Michigan: Servant Publications, 1991), p. 190.

2. John Bradshaw, *Family Secrets* (New York: Ballantine Books, 1995), p. 274.

Recommended Reading

MIND-BODY HEALTH

Benson, Herbert, M.D., with Marg Stark, *Timeless Healing: The Power and Biology of Belief.* New York: Scribner, 1996.

Chopra, Deepak, M.D., *Ageless Body, Timeless Mind.* New York: Harmony Books, 1993.

Dacher, Elliott S., M.D., *PNI-Psychoneuroimmunology: The Mind/Body Healing Program.* New York: Paragon House, 1991.

Goleman, Daniel, *Emotional Intelligence.* New York: Bantam Books, 1995.

Hay, Louise L., *You Can Heal Your Life.* Farmingdale, New York: Coleman Publishing, 1984.

Levine, Barbara Hoberman, *Your Body Believes Every Word You Say.* Lower Lake, California: Azlan Publishing, 1991.

Mason, L. John, Ph.D., *Stress Passages.* Berkeley, California: Celestial Arts, 1988.

Mehl, Lewis E., M.D., Ph.D., *Mind and Matter: A Healing Approach to Chronic Illness.* Berkeley, California: Mind/Body Press, 1986.

Minirth, Frank, M.D., *The Power of Memories: How to Use Them to Improve Your Health and Well-Being.* Nashville, Tennessee: Thomas Nelson Publishers, 1995.

Naparstek, Belleruth, *Staying Well With Guided Imagery: How to Harness the Power of Your Imagination for Health and Healing.* New York: Warner Books, 1994.

Northrup, Christiane, M.D., *Women's Bodies, Women's Wisdom: Creating Physical and Emotional Health and Healing.* New York: Bantam Books, 1994.

Peper, Erik, Sonia Ancoli, and Michele Quinn, *Mind/Body Integration.* New York: Plenum Press, 1979.

Rossi, Ernest, *The Psychobiology of Mind-Body Healing.* New York: W. W. Norton, 1986.

Williams, Redford, M.D., and Virginia Williams, Ph.D., *Anger Kills.* New York: Harper-Collins, 1993.

REPRODUCTION

Fleming, Anne Taylor, *Motherhood Deferred: A Woman's Journey*. New York: Fawcett Columbine, 1994.

Harkness, Carla, *The Infertility Book: A Comprehensive Medical & Emotional Guide*. Berkeley, California: Celestial Arts, 1992.

Scher, Jonathan, M.D., and Carol Dix, *Preventing Miscarriage: The Good News*. New York: HarperCollins, 1991.

Simons, Harriet Fishman, *Wanting Another Child: Coping With Secondary Infertility*. New York: Simon & Schuster, 1995.

Vaughan, Christopher, *How Life Begins: The Science of Life in the Womb*. New York: Random House, 1996.

Verny, Thomas, M.D., with John Kelly, *The Secret Life of the Unborn Child*. New York: Bantam, Doubleday, Dell Publishing, 1981.

WOMEN'S ISSUES

Edelman, Hope, *Motherless Daughters*. New York: Bantam, Doubleday, Dell Publishing, 1994.

Estés, Clarissa Pinkola, Ph.D., *Women Who Run with the Wolves: Myths and Stories of the Wild Woman Archetype*. New York: Ballantine Books, 1992.

Hochschild, Arlie, with Anne Machung, *The Second Shift*. New York: Avon Books, 1989.

Leonard, Linda Schierse, *The Wounded Woman: Healing the Father-Daughter Relationship*. Boston: Shambhala, 1992.

Lerner, Harriet G., Ph.D., *The Dance of Anger*. New York: Harper & Row, 1985.

Maine, Margo, Ph.D., *Father Hunger: Fathers, Daughters & Food*. Carlsburg, California: Gurze Books, 1991.

McBroom, Patricia A., *The Third Sex: The New Professional Woman*. New York: Paragon House, 1992.

Murdock, Maureen, *Fathers' Daughters: Transforming the Father-Daughter Relationship*. New York: Ballantine, 1994.

Rivers, Caryl, Rosalind Barnett, and Grace Baruch, *How Women Grow, Learn & Thrive*. New York: Ballantine Books, 1979.

Wakerman, Elyce, *Father Loss*. New York: Henry Holt, 1984.

MEN'S ISSUES

Allen, Marvin, with Jo Robinson, *Angry Men, Passive Men*. New York: Fawcett Columbine, 1993.

Osherson, Samuel, *Finding Our Fathers: How a Man's Life Is Shaped by His Relationship With His Father*. New York: Fawcett Columbine, 1986.

Pittman, Frank, M.D., *Man Enough: Fathers, Sons, and the Search for Masculinity*. New York: Berkley Publishing, 1993.

Shapiro, Jerrold Lee, Ph.D., *The Measure of Man*. New York: Berkley Publishing, 1993.

LOVE RELATIONSHIPS

Hendrix, Harville, Ph.D., *Getting the Love You Want*. New York: Harper & Row, 1988.

Maslin, Bonnie, Ph.D., *The Angry Marriage: Overcoming the Rage, Reclaiming the Love*. New York: Hyperion, 1994.

Mason, L. John, *Stress Passages*. Berkeley, California: Celestial Arts, 1988.

Wade, Brenda, Ph.D. and Brenda Lane Richardson, *Love Lessons: A Guide to Transforming Relationships*. New York: Amistad Books, 1993.

Welwood, John, Ph.D., *Journey of the Heart: Intimate Relationships and the Path of Love*. New York: HarperCollins Publishers, 1990.

GENERAL PSYCHOLOGY

Ackroyd, Eric, *A Dictionary of Dream Symbols: With an Introduction to Dream Psychology*. New York: Sterling Publishing Co., 1993.

Borysenko, Joan, Ph.D., *Guilt Is the Teacher, Love Is the Lesson*. New York: Warner Books, 1990.

Conger, John P., Ph.D., *Jung & Reich: The Body as Shadow*. Berkeley, California: North Atlantic Books, 1988.

— — —, *The Body in Recovery*. Berkeley, California: Frog, Ltd., 1994.

Engel, Lewis, Ph.D., and Tom Ferguson, M.D., *Hidden Guilt: How to Stop Punishing Yourself and Enjoy the Happiness You Deserve*. New York: Pocket Books, 1990.

Fishel, Elizabeth, *I Swore I'd Never Do That: Recognizing Family Patterns & Making Wise Parenting Choices*. Emeryville, California: Conari Press, 1991.

Foster, Carolyn, *The Family Patterns Workbook: Breaking Free From Your Past and Creating a Life of Your Own*. New York: Jeremy P. Tarcher/Perigee, 1993.

Golomb, Elan, Ph.D., *Trapped in the Mirror: Adult Children of Narcissists in Their Struggle for Self*. New York: William Morrow and Company, Inc., 1992.

Hoffman, Bob, *No One Is to Blame: Freedom from Compulsive Self-defeating Behavior*. Oakland, California: Recycling Books, 1988.

Love, Dr. Patricia, with Jo Robinson, *The Emotional Incest Syndrome: What to Do When a Parent's Love Rules Your Life*. New York: Bantam Books, 1990.

Martin, April, Ph.D., *Lesbian & Gay Parenting Handbook*. New York: HarperCollins, 1993.

Minuchin, Salvador, *Families & Family Therapy*. Cambridge, Massachusetts: Harvard University Press, 1974.

Peck, M. Scott, M.D., *The Road Less Traveled: A New Psychology of Love, Traditional Values and Spiritual Growth*. New York: Simon & Schuster, 1978.

Stoop, Dr. David, and Dr. James Masteller, *Forgiving Our Parents, Forgiving Ourselves*. Ann Arbor, Michigan: Servant Publications, 1991.

Walker, Alice, *The Untouched Key: Tracing Childhood Trauma in Creativity and Destructiveness*. New York: Bantam, 1990.

Weinberg, Dr. George, *Society and the Healthy Homosexual: How to Get the Most Out of Being Gay*. Boston: Alyson Publications, 1972.

Whitfield, Charles L., M.D. *Healing the Child Within*. Deerfield Beach, Florida: Health Communications, Inc., 1987.

Zweig, Connie, and Jeremiah Abrams, *Meeting the Shadow: The Hidden Power of the Dark Side of Human Nature*. Los Angeles: Jeremy P. Tarcher, Inc., 1991.

SIBLING RELATIONSHIPS

Greer, Dr. Jane, *Adult Sibling Rivalry*. New York: Ballantine Books, 1992.

Klagsbrun, Francine, *Mixed Feelings: Love, Hate, Rivalry, and Reconciliation Among Brothers and Sisters*. New York: Bantam Books, 1992.

Mathias, Barbara, *Between Sisters*. New York: Dell Publishing, 1992.

SOCIAL PERSPECTIVES

Asbell, Bernard, *The Pill: A Biography of the Drug That Changed the World*. New York: Random House, 1995.

Cose, Ellis, *The Rage of a Privileged Class*. New York: Harper Collins, 1993.

Sheehy, Gail, *New Passages: Mapping Your Life Across Time*. New York: Random House, 1995.

Resources

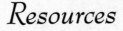

Niravi B. Payne, M.S.
Whole Person Fertility Program^{SM}
100 Remsen Street
Brooklyn, NY 11201
For a referral roster of Whole Person Fertility Program^{SM} therapists or for a schedule of training courses, please call 800-666-HEALTH or 718-625-4802 or e-mail niravi@aol.com.

Mind/Body Tension/Relax Biofeedback Card
Contact: Renia Norflis
Optimal Health Associates
100 Remsen Street
Brooklyn, NY 11201
800-666-HEALTH
Please send $2.50 + 50¢ postage.

"Nature's Ode to Conception" tape by Niravi B. Payne, M.S.
Optimal Health Associates
100 Remsen Street
Brooklyn, NY 11201
$10.00 + $1.00 postage (please make checks payable to Niravi B. Payne, M.S.)

Christiane Northrup, M.D.
Health Wisdom for Women
Phillips Publishing, Inc.
P.O. Box 60042
7811 Montrose Road
Potomac, MD 20859-0042
800-221-8561

Marcelle Pick, M.S.N., R.N.G., OB/GYN and
Pediatric, N.P., Owner/Director
Women to Women
1 Pleasant Street
Yarmouth, ME 04096
207-846-6163

Bethany Hays, M.D., F.A.C.O.G.
Women to Women
1 Pleasant Street
Yarmouth, ME 04096
207-846-6163

Allan Warshowsky, M.D., F.A.C.O.G.
Holistic OB/GYN
2001 Marcus Avenue
New Hyde Park, NY 11042
516-488-2757

Both Dr. Hays and Dr. Warshowsky have an obstetrical/gynecological practice with a strong holistic mind-body approach encouraging women to take charge of their health care.

Jonathan Scher, M.D.
1126 Park Avenue
New York, NY 10128
212-427-7400
Author of Preventing Miscarriages.

Hoffman Institute
223 San Anselmo Avenue
Suite 4
San Anselmo, CA 94960
415-485-5220

RESOLVE, Inc.
1310 Broadway
Somerville, MA 02144-1731
617-623-1156
Helpline: 617-623-0744

American Holistic Medical Association
4101 Lake Boone Trail
Raleigh, NC 27607
919-787-5181

American Society for Reproductive Medicine
1209 Montgomery Highway
Birmingham, AL 35216-2809
205-978-5000

Joan Borysenko, Ph.D.
Mind-Body Health Sciences, Inc.
393 Dixon Road
Boulder, CO 80302
303-440-8460

Tamara Slayton
Menstrual Health Foundation
WomanKind
P.O. Box 1775
Sebastopol, CA 95473
707-522-8662
Fax 707-579-6229
As a reflection of changing attitudes, this organization is supporting women and girls as they celebrate their periods through rituals and workshops.

BOOKS

Healing into Life and Death, the "Womb Meditation" chapter, by Stephen Levine (New York: Anchor Books/Doubleday, 1987).

Preventing Miscarriage by Jonathan Scher and Carol Dix (New York: HarperCollins, 1991).

Stress Passages by L. John Mason (Berkeley, California: Celestial Arts, 1988). Offers information about tension, visualizations, sexual functions, and massage. For audiotapes, write to L. John Mason, 315 East Cotati Avenue, Suite F, Cotati, CA 94931 or call 707-795-2228.

Index